Melba Wilson was born in Virginia, USA and raised in Texas. Based in London since 1977, she is a freelance journalist writing on health and social issues relating to Britain's black communities, with particular reference to black women.

Her articles, reviews and essays have been published in *New Society*, *Feminist Review*, *City Limits* and *Africa* magazine. She has contributed to several anthologies including *Why Children?* (Women's Press, 1980), *Charting the Journey: Writing by Black and Third World Women* (Sheba Feminist Publishers, 1987) and *Feminism and Censorship* (Prism Press, 1988). She is author of *Crossing the Boundary: Black Women Survive Incest* (Virago, 1993).

Active in the black women's movement in Britain and internationally, Melba Wilson is married with two children.

Healthy and Wise

*The Essential Health Handbook
For Black Women*

Edited by Melba Wilson

Acknowledgements

....

Permission to reproduce the following material is gratefully acknowledged: 'Sick and Tired of Being Sick and Tired: The Politics of Black Women's Health' reproduced from *Women, Culture and Politics* by Angela Y. Davis; and 'Beauty: When the Other Dancer is the Self' reproduced from *In Search of Our Mother's Gardens* by Alice Walker both are published in Great Britain by The Women's Press Ltd, 34 Great Sutton Street, London EC1V 0DX. 'Prescriptions of Root Doctors' from *Mules and Men* by Zora Neale Hurston. Copyright © 1935 by Zora Neal Hurston. Copyright renewed 1963 by John C. Hurston and Joel Hurston. Reprinted by permission of HarperCollins, Publishers, Inc. 'Taking the Home Out of Homophobia: Black Lesbian Health' by Jewelle L. Gomez and Barbara Smith from *The Black Womans Health Book* edited by Evelyn C. White, reproduced by kind permission of Seal Press, Seattle, USA. 'Living With Cancer' from *A Burst of Light* by Audre Lorde, reproduced by kind permission of Sheba Feminist Press, 10a Bradbury Street, London N16 8JN. The illustration 'The Pump' on p233 is reproduced from *Reclaim Your Power* by Khaleghl Quinn by kind permission of Thorsons Publishers, London. Lines from 'Black Brown White Blues' by William Broonzy copyright © Duchess Music Corporation reproduced with kind permission of MCA Music Ltd.

Published by VIRAGO PRESS Limited, April 1994
42–43 Gloucester Crescent, London NW1 7PD

*A CIP catalogue record for this title
is available from the British Library*

Typeset by Florencetype Ltd, Kewstoke, Avon
Printed in Great Britain by
Cox & Wyman Ltd, Reading, Berkshire

Contents

···

Introduction

Melba Wilson

When we think about health, it is easy to restrict our consideration to a narrow definition. We tend to regard the state of our health as a very private or individual thing. We may worry about the odd ache or pain, or may view our health in terms of whether we are eating too much, drinking too much or becoming too stressed out. We may *not* worry about our health. We may tend to think, as we so often do when we are young, that we are invincible and that somehow neither illness nor infirmity will touch us.

If we are black and female, we are more likely to be in the latter category, simply because we cannot afford or don't see how we can take the time to dwell on our own health. More often than not, this is due to the fact that we are so busy tending to the needs – health and otherwise – of others that there really isn't the time. If and when we *are* forced to deal with our own health needs, it may be at the point of crisis or within the context of making do with inadequate or insensitive services, or of trying to call upon our own reserves or energies to tackle what ails us. In the main, this is undertaken very much within an individualised framework, and we often fail to make the connections between the state of our health and the effects of societal factors upon it.

It is important to say, however, and it is a strand which runs throughout the work of the women who contribute to this book, that the health of black people, and black women especially, cannot be looked at in isolation from our position as black people within a racist society or indeed, without recognising the strengths which we, as people of colour, can bring to an informed assessment of black people's health needs. In 'Sick and Tired of Being Sick and Tired' Angela Davis put it this way:

> We have become cognisant of the urgency of contextualising Black women's health in relation to the prevailing political conditions. While our health is undeniably assaulted by natural forces frequently beyond our control, all too often the enemies of our physical and emotional well-being are social and political. That is why we must strive to understand the complex politics of Black women's health.

Any discussion concerning black women's health is at once personal and political. By definition, it must also be practical. Personal in the sense that we owe it to ourselves to establish a familiarity with our bodies, our psyches, in order that we are better able to understand, interpret, react to or, better still, anticipate the messages that come to us about our own health requirements. Political in the sense that, at the same time, we must come to the realisation that health is not a concept to be looked at within a vacuum, nor is it one over which we have sole control. Instead, it is influenced by environmental and social factors which have direct links to health concerns. The practicalities of good health and good health care require that as black people, we intervene in the health care system to inform policy and practice, and in so doing safeguard our interests in the benefits which flow from that system. To divorce any one aspect – the personal, political or practical – from the other is to leave ourselves open, as communities and people of colour, to remaining vulnerable, in terms of access to health care, as well as in gaining an understanding of what our needs are and how to articulate them within the wider community.

But what does it mean to discuss health in a political perspective? Surely, health *is* an individual matter, many would argue. Are we not, after all, responsible for our own health and social welfare? Is it not directly within our own control?

Well, the answer must be no, not exactly. Often as black people we do not have the information we need to make informed decisions about our health care. We may have difficulty negotiating the health care system; we may be intimidated by members of the medical profession who take umbrage at any attempts to question their practice or (perhaps more pertinently when it comes to black people) malpractice. We do not have access to funds which could stimulate research into health services geared towards meeting the specific needs of black people, for example research into sickle cell anaemia. And finally, we do not, in the main, have access to the decision-making channels – national government, district health authorities, community health councils – which decide how, where and towards whom health resources are prioritised and directed.

Within this scenario the specific health needs and concerns of women generally, as a sub-group of the total population, with a stake in such resources, are not generally recognised or acted upon. When we look at the position of black women the gap between needs being met in a culturally sensitive manner and the consequent targeting of resources – including appropriate personnel as well as financial resources – widens even further.

In 1978 the then Department of Health and Social Security issued a circular . . . following the 1976 Race Relations Act, which called on health authorities to implement 'effective positive procedures to ensure equality of opportunity'. In 1988, the National Association of Health Authorities

(NAHA) convened a working party which produced *Action not words*, a strategy to improve health services for Black and minority ethnic groups. The report defined what the working group understood by equality in the NHS. This definition included a statement that all people irrespective of their religion, culture, race, colour or ethnic background should have equal access to the NHS, services relevant to their needs, be treated with respect when using health services, have equal access to employment in the NHS and have equal rights of representation on health authorities, community health councils and other agencies.[1]

The latest additions to the legislation, reports and provision for services affecting Britain's black communities are the Health of the Nation initiative launched in 1992, the NHS and Community Care Act 1990 and the Children Act 1989. All have as part of their stated objectives the bringing about of greater access to health and social services for black people; and both specifically emphasise the importance of considering racial origin and cultural and linguistic background in service delivery.

The reality for black people, on the whole, is that we are pushed even nearer to the margins of health service delivery. This is due to a combination of factors. The internal market of the NHS, with increasingly restricted and finite budgets, means that prioritised needs are the order of the day. Given that black people's health needs have traditionally been under- or ill-considered, it is even more important to ensure that our voices are heard. The planned closure of a number of hospitals in inner London, recently announced by Health Secretary Virginia Bottomley, is a case in point. The closure of health facilities in the communities where we live will exacerbate the problems that black people already have in gaining access to what is, even now, limited health care. In addition, the lack of adequate funding for community care means that more and more people will receive either no care or inappropriate care, as

in the case of black people being disproportionately insti-
tutionalised as a result of mental illness diagnoses.

The overriding consideration for black people within all
of this, of course, must be the institutional racism which
confronts us as we try to get the system to respond to our
needs. Institutional racism is found for example, in the failure to prioritise the needs of black elders, because of the
prevailing attitude that we look after our own. It is found
in the colour-blind approach to service delivery, which
treats everyone the same and tries to ignore the effects of
racism and discrimination in housing, education and
employment in black people's lives. It is to be found in
practice which tends to treat black people with the heavy
hand of the medical model (as in the use of psychiatric
institutions and drugs, rather than therapeutic alternatives),
with little regard for exploring more culturally appropriate
methods of treatment or of listening to what black people
themselves have to say about their health needs.

In arguing the need for a new perspective on black
women's health, specifically in relation to HIV and AIDS,
for example, Patricia January-Bardill notes in her chapter
that: 'an analysis of the state of health of any society
must include health education, nutrition, mental health,
the organisation of health care as well as the impact of
social, economic, political, ideological and legal systems'.
She adds however, and unsurprisingly that: 'Black women
do not control the institutions that affect their health and
well being. On the contrary, the objective social reality of
black women is that they are at the bottom of the social
pecking order in the UK.'

The aim of this book is to contribute to the amount of
information which is available to black people, and black
women in particular, to enable us to make more informed
choices and decisions concerning our health needs. I have
used a very broad definition of health in compiling the
book, as can be seen from the range of subjects it covers.

All of us speak with one voice in approaching health in its totality – looking not just at physical manifestations, but at emotional, cultural and societal influences as well.

It is incumbent upon us all, as black people, to work towards the concept of good health care which is accessible and equitable for all. In order to do this we need tools which can aid this process. The women who have contributed to this book bring a wealth of information and expertise from their respective fields. The body of work which makes up this book goes some way in providing those tools.

Melba Wilson
1994

Note
1. Greater London Association of Community Health Councils, 'Proposal for a project on CHCs/Race and ethnicity', September 1992.

Sick and Tired of Being Sick and Tired: the Politics of Black Women's Health★

Angela Y. Davis

Politics do not stand in polar opposition to our lives. Whether we desire it or not, they permeate our existence, insinuating themselves into the most private spaces of our lives. As a starting point for this discussion of the politics of Black women's health, I propose we consider the lived experience of one courageous individual who, as she poignantly documents her own personal health battles, harvests lessons that elucidate our collective quest for wellness. 'How do I provide myself,' Audre Lorde asks,

> with the best physical and psychic nourishment to repair past, and minimize future damage to my body? How do I give voice to my quests so that other women can take what they need from my experiences? How do my experiences with cancer fit into the larger tapestry of my work as a Black woman, into the history of all women? And most of all, how do I fight the despair born of fear and anger and powerlessness which is my greatest internal enemy?
>
> I have found that battling despair does not mean closing my eyes to the enormity of the tasks of effecting change, nor

★This address was first given in August 1987 at Bennett College, Greensboro, North Carolina, before a conference organised by the North Carolina Black Women's Health Project. As Davis tells it, it is time for black women to fight back on every front and reclaim our health.

ignoring the strength and the barbarity of the forces aligned against us. It means teaching, surviving and fighting with the most important resource I have, myself, and taking joy in that battle. It means, for me, recognizing the enemy outside and the enemy within, and knowing that my work is part of a continuum of women's work, of reclaiming this earth and our power, and knowing that this work did not begin with my birth nor will it end with my death. And it means knowing that within this continuum, my life and my love and my work has particular power and meaning relative to others.

It means trout fishing on the Missisquoi River at dawn and tasting the green silence, and knowing that this beauty too is mine forever.[1]

On this continuum of women's work, upon which Audre Lorde situates herself and her precious offerings, the pursuit of health in body, mind and spirit weaves in and out of every major struggle women have ever waged in our quest for social, economic and political emancipation. During the past decade we have been the fortunate beneficiaries of the valuable work of health activists like Byllye Avery and Lillie Allen of the National Black Women's Health Project, who have perceptively and passionately addressed Black women's health issues and have begun to chart out paths toward wellness in all its myriad forms. The Project has chosen as its motto Fannie Lou Hamer's well-known lament: We are sick and tired of being sick and tired.

We have become cognisant of the urgency of contextualising Black women's health in relation to the prevailing political conditions. While our health is undeniably assaulted by natural forces frequently beyond our control, all too often the enemies of our physical and emotional well-being are social and political. That is why we must strive to understand the complex politics of Black women's health.

One would assume that the US Constitution, which guarantees all individuals 'life, liberty and the pursuit of happiness', by implication assures that all citizens of that country are entitled to be healthy. However, it is not really necessary to derive this right from the Constitution, for health ought to be universally recognised as a basic human right. Yet in American society, dominated as it is by the profit-seeking ventures of monopoly corporations, health has been callously transformed into a commodity – a commodity that those with means are able to afford, but that is too often entirely beyond the reach of others. Pregnant Black women, uninsured and without the means to pay hospital entrance fees, have been known to give birth in parking lots outside the hospitals that have refused them entry. In other instances, poor Black women who are subscribers to health plans have been denied treatment because hospital officials have presumptuously argued that they were lying about their insurance coverage.

Sharon Ford, a young Black woman on welfare in the San Francisco Bay area, gave birth to a stillborn child because two hospitals declined to treat her, even though she was covered by a health plan. Aware of a serious problem with her pregnancy, Ms Ford sought treatment at the hospital nearest her home. When she informed officials there that she was covered by a certain medical plan, she was sent by them to the hospital associated with that plan, despite the fact that her critical condition obviously warranted emergency intervention. Officials at the second hospital, who claimed that their computerised list of subscribers to that plan did not include her name, instructed her to go to yet another facility, known as the poor people's medical warehouse in that area. In the meantime, however, three hours had passed, and by the time she was treated by doctors at the third hospital, her unborn baby had died. Ironically, it was later discovered that the insurance company had been tardy in delivering the subscriber list that, indeed, contained Sharon Ford's name. While this is the tragic story of a single Black woman, it cannot be dismissed as an aberration. Rather, it is symptomatic of dangerous trends within the health care industry.

Because so many programmes designed to ameliorate the conditions of poor people – inadequate as they may have been – have been abolished or cut back in recent years, accessibility to health services has become an especially pressing problem. The major barrier to Black women's health is poverty – and during the Reagan years our communities became increasingly impoverished. The number of poor people increased by more than 6 million, and according to the Physicians' Task Force on Hunger, as many as 20 million people in this country suffered from want of food. A dire consequence of poverty is malnutrition and a plethora of diseases emanating from the lack of adequate sustenance. Malnutrition, which can cause maternal anaemia and toxaemia, a potentially fatal condition for a pregnant woman, is also implicated in premature births and infant deaths.

Associated with higher rates of chronic illnesses such as heart disease, arthritis and diabetes, poverty causes its victims to be more susceptible to hypertension and lung, stomach and oesophageal cancer. The National Black Women's Health Project has pointed out that while proportionately fewer Black women than white women suffer from breast cancer, more Black women are likely to die from it. Furthermore, as cervical cancer rates have decreased among white women, they have risen among Black women. For reasons that require no explanation, poverty increases vulnerability to mental illness. Of all groups in the US, Black women have the highest rates of admission to outpatient psychiatric services. It has been argued by health activists that most adult Black women live in a state of psychological stress.

Two out of three poor adults are women, and 80 per cent of the poor in the United States are women and children. This means that women are the majority of the recipients of many health and nutritional programmes sponsored by the federal government. Because Black women are disproportionately represented among the beneficiaries of these social services, they have been hurt most deeply by the cutbacks in the federal budget. When the cutbacks in Aid to Families with Dependent Children (AFDC) occurred, most of the women who lost AFDC also lost their Medicaid coverage. Federal cuts in the Maternal and Child Health Block Grant resulted, in almost all states, in the reduction of services offered in maternal and child health clinics, or in the curtailment of the number of people eligible to receive this care. As a consequence, almost a million people, most of whom are children and women of childbearing age, became ineligible to receive services at community health centres. This means, for example, that fewer Black women now receive prenatal care, a fact that has fatal implications, because babies born to mothers receiving no prenatal care are three times more likely to die in infancy than those whose mothers do receive such care. At the same time, federal funding for abortions has become virtually nonexistent, while the government continues to strongly subsidise surgical sterilisation. This process is a vicious cycle, further entrenching poor people in conditions that make ill-health inevitable. Standing at the intersection of racism, sexism and economic injustice, Black women have been compelled to bear the brunt of this complex oppressive process.

Afro-American women are twice as likely as white women to die of hypertensive cardiovascular disease, and they have three times the rate of high blood pressure. Black infant mortality is twice that of whites, and maternal mortality is three times as high. Lupus is three times more common among Black women than white, so the funds channelled into research to discover a cure for it have been extremely sparse. Far more Black than white women die as a result of diabetes and cancer.

This cycle of oppression is largely responsible for the fact that far too many Black women resort to drugs as a means – however ineffective it ultimately proves to be – of softening the blows of poverty. Because of intravenous drug use in the Black community, a disproportionately large number of Black women have been infected with AIDS. Although the popular belief is that AIDS is a disease of gay white men, the truth is that Afro-Americans and Latinos are far more likely to contract AIDS than whites. This is true among gays, among IV drug users, among hetero-sexual partners, and among children. Black and Latino men are two and a half times as likely to get AIDS as white men. Latina women are nine times as likely as white women to contract AIDS. But the most frightening statistic is reserved for Black women, who are twelve times more likely than white women to contract the AIDS virus.

Four times as many Black women as white women die of homicide. In the meantime, under the Reagan adminis-tration, hospitals serving predominantly poor Black communities – including those with excellent trauma units, designed to treat victims of violence – closed down. Such was the case with the Homer G. Phillips Hospital in St Louis, the largest teaching hospital for Black medical students in the USA. On average in this country, there is one doctor per 1,500 people, but in central Harlem there is only one doctor per 4,500 people.

A statement by the Public Health Association of New York City during the first year of the Reagan administra-tion warned:

The health of the people of New York City is actively endangered by the already imposed cuts and by the threatened cuts in funding for health care services and for medical care services. To express ourselves in clear language, so there is no misunderstanding: We are talking about dead babies whose death can be prevented; we are talking about sick children and adults whose illnesses can be prevented; we are talking about misery for older people whose misery can be prevented. We are speaking of these unspeakable things in a wealthy country and in a wealthy state, whose people deserve better. The malignant neglect of federal, state and local governments is literally killing people now and will kill and destroy the lives of many more in the future. We urge a massive infusion of federal and state funds to restore and rebuild services now, before the consequences of their breakdown demonstrate in even more tragic and dramatic ways the human and economic cost of this neglect.[2]

Outside of South Africa, the United States is the only major industrial country in the world that lacks a uniform national health insurance plan. While this country is sorely in need of a national health care plan, there has been an increasing trend towards the privatisation of health care. As one book plainly put it, the principle of the Reagan administration was 'Profits Before People, Greed Before Need, and Wealth Before Health'.[3]

In urging the privatisation of health care, the government has prioritised the profit-seeking interests of monopoly corporations, leaving the health needs of poor people – and especially poor Black women – to be callously juggled around and, when need be, ignored. For-profit hospitals often refuse outright to treat poor, uninsured patients, and they engage in the unethical practice of 'dumping' welfare recipients on public hospitals, even when those patients are in urgent need of treatment. This was the unfortunate fate of Sharon Ford, whose baby became one of the many fatalities of a process that places profits before people's health needs.

Because the hospital emergency room is a major setting for medical treatment in the Black community, this pattern of the privatisation of hospitals is having an especially devastating impact on Black people – and on Black women in particular. In 1983 only 44.1 per cent of Afro-Americans receiving health care made visits to a private doctor in her or his office. On the other hand, 26.5 per cent went to a hospital emergency room and 9.7 per cent received treatment in an outpatient clinic. By contrast, 57 per cent of white patients receiving medical care visited private physicians, 13 per cent went to emergency rooms and 16 per cent to outpatient clinics.

The degree to which private corporations threaten to monopolise health care services is revealed by the fact that the Hospital Corporation of America, which controlled two hospitals in 1968, now controls almost 500 and is a dominant force in the hospital business. Other such corporations are Cigna, American Medical International and Humana. Health care workers – a majority of whom are women in the lower-paying occupations – have also suffered from this privatisation trend, for corporate takeovers of public hospitals have frequently resulted in union-busting and a subsequent freeze on wages and cutbacks on benefits.

> The only ones who benefit from a competition system of medical care are the rich, who will have to pay less for health care for the poor, and those providers who skim the cream off the medical market and leave the real problems to a diminished and even-more-inadequately-financed public sector. It is yet another example of the basic Reagan policy of serving the rich, encased in a Trojan Horse, this one labelled 'cost containment,' 'deregulation,' and 'free choice.'[4]

It is clearly in the interests of Afro-American women to demand a federally subsidised, uniform national health insurance plan. We need subsidised programmes that reflect the progressive experiences of the women's health movement over the last decade and a half, programmes that emphasise prevention, self-help and empowerment.

One of the main obstacles to the development of a national health plan is the same unrelenting pressure placed by the US government on all social programmes benefiting poor people, and people of colour in particular – namely, the runaway military budget. Since 1980 the military budget has more than doubled, taking approximately $100 billion from social programmes that were underfunded to begin with. Between 1981 and 1986, $1.5 trillion was spent on military programmes. As the Women's International League for Peace and Freedom points out:

> Defense Department spending in 1986 was $292 billion, but the actual costs of the military in that year were over $400 billion if hidden costs like veterans benefits, nuclear warheads in the Department of Energy's budget, and the part of the interest on the national debt attributable to past military expenditures are taken into account.[5]

The budget cuts that have affected health and other social services are not, strictly speaking, cuts, but rather transfers of funds from the civilian to the military budget. Instead of providing poor people with adequate food stamps, the corporations that make up the military-industrial complex are awarded gigantic defence contracts. Ironically, forty-five of the top one hundred defence contractors who received more than $100 billion in prime-contract awards in 1985 later came under criminal investigation.[6]

As we examine the political forces responsible for the violation of Black women's health rights in the US, it becomes clear that the increasing militarisation of the economy is culpable in a major way. The politics of Black women's health are also directly influenced by the general assault on democracy in this country, which reached a high point during the Reagan years. It is not a coincidence that a government that would sabotage the rights of every citizen by permitting the development of a secret junta controlled by the Central Intelligence Agency and the National Security Council also seriously infringed the health rights of Black women and all poor people.

The Iran-Contra hearings revealed the extent to which we were rapidly heading in the direction of a police state. The CIA operatives involved used government and private funds to support the most reactionary forces in the world – from the Contras in Nicaragua to the South-African-supported UNITA in Angola. They were involved in gun running, drug trafficking, bombings, assassinations, and attempted overthrows of democratically elected governments.

The executive branch of the government during the Reagan years was dominated by corporate executives and by top military men. They continued to serve the monopoly corporations as they carried out the bellicose policies of the military. As they conducted undeclared wars in various parts of the world, they were responsible for the domestic war against poor people, one of whose battlefields involved the cutbacks in health services whose effects have been so detrimental to Black women.

Reagan's 1987 nomination of the ultraconservative Robert Bork to the Supreme Court was yet another offensive against the welfare of Black women and others who suffer from racism, sexism and economic exploitation. As Senator Edward Kennedy so poignantly observed, 'Robert Bork's America is a land in which women would be forced into back-alley abortions, Blacks would sit down at segregated lunch counters, [and] rogue police would break down citizens' doors in midnight raids.' Fortunately, progressive forces joined hands and succeeded in blocking the confirmation of Judge Bork to the Supreme Court.

It is from the success of progressive campaigns such as this one, as well as from the important work of organisations such as the National Black Women's Health Project, that all of us who are concerned with remedying the deplorable state of health care in this country must glean important lessons. We must learn consistently to place our battle for universally accessible health care in its larger social and political context. We must recognise the importance of raising our voices in opposition to such backward forces as Robert Bork and the outdated conservatism he represents. We must involve ourselves in the anti-apartheid movement in solidarity with our sisters and brothers in South Africa, who not only suffer the ill effects of negligent health care but are daily murdered in cold blood by the South African government. We must actively oppose the US government's continuing bid for Congressional support of Contra aid; we must not allow our sisters and brothers in Nicaragua, whose revolutionary strivings have made health care available to all of their country's inhabitants on an equal basis, to be defeated.

While we fight for these larger victories, we must also learn to applaud the small victories we win. As I opened with the wise words of Audre Lorde, so I would like to conclude with this passage taken from her book, *A Burst of Light*:

> Battling racism and battling heterosexism and battling apartheid share the same urgency inside me as battling cancer. None of these struggles is ever easy, and even the smallest victory must be applauded, because it is so easy not to battle at all, to just accept, and to call that acceptance inevitable.[7]

Notes

1. Audre Lorde, *The Cancer Journals*, San Francisco, Spinsters/Aunt Lute, 1980, p. 17.
2. Alan Gartner, Colin Greer and Frank Riessman, *What Reagan is Doing to Us*, New York, Harper & Row, 1982, p. 50.
3. Ibid., p. 48.
4. Ibid., p. 46.
5. 'The Women's Budget', Women's International League For Peace and Freedom, 1986, p. 3.
6. Ibid.
7. Audre Lorde, *A Burst of Light*, Ithaca, NY, Firebrand Books, 1988, pp. 116–17.

Black Women and Health: a Political Overview of British Health Care

Protasia Torkington

There is still a general tendency to perceive health as peripheral to major social, political and economic issues; to view ill-health as something that people must face individually, when they or their relatives and friends fall ill or die. More often than not, lip service is paid to the frequently quoted phrase, 'Health is a political issue'. What is even more depressing is when health is given a low or no priority at all in conferences or discourses that are specifically concerned with women's experiences. Health issues are central to our life.

My conviction about the centrality of health in women's lives is not only an academic interest but also arises from practical involvement in the field. I have worked as an employee in both South Africa and England. I have spent a considerable amount of my academic life conducting research in the National Health Service as well as teaching on courses concerned with health issues. My major involvement, however, is not as an employee or researcher but as a user, and it is from this position that I share with many other women the oppressive aspects of the health service.

Many who are critical of the NHS acknowledge that the system has had some advantages for the British public in general. At the point of delivery, health care has been free for all, which has meant that even those who were not able to pay National Insurance contributions were not left without treatment. However, this positive aspect has been undermined by the role medicine has played as a form of social control. While this is true in relation to all users, that control is more sharply felt by women: for a number of reasons women tend to have more interaction with the health professionals who implement that process of social control.

Firstly, the biological and anatomical constitution of women means that we can suffer from additional illnesses such as breast cancer, cervical cancer, ovarian cysts, salpingitis and many more that men do not experience. Secondly, even when women go through normal, natural processes of pregnancy and childbirth, these have been so medicalised that interaction with health professionals is now a matter of course. Equally, there is no escape for hetero-sexual women who do not want to have children because the dominant forms of contraception, such as the pill, intra-uterine devices and sterilisation, are controlled and administered by health professionals. Thirdly, the unequal division of labour within the family means that women tend to look after children and elderly relatives. When these dependants fall ill it is women who take them for consultation to health professionals. Some women who have found their male partners helpful with this task have nevertheless pointed out that men sometimes come back with such confused and garbled information about what the doctor said or prescribed that the women felt it would have been better to have gone with the relative in the first place. Fourthly, when some men fall ill they still have a tendency to maintain the 'stiff upper lip' and avoid taking medical advice during the early stages of an illness. Sometimes consultation is put off until the condition is so bad that women end up having to accompany their partners or risk the accusation of being unloving and uncaring.

Within the health service the most dominant group with which women interact is the medical profession (doctors, nurses and so on). Within that group there is 'the belief that women are essentially reproductive and ultimately inferior'.[1] The medical ideology which fosters this belief is a reflection of the sexism which exists in the wider social, political and economic structure. To a large extent, women's proper contribution to society is still believed to be within the domestic sphere as housewives and mothers. There is evidence that women who challenge this stereotype may run the risk of being labelled abnormal or, in some cases, mentally ill. The experience of Barbara, as related by one speaker at a conference, illustrates the dilemma faced by women in this area. Barbara hated doing housework and this was the source of many rows with her husband Tom. Tom could not see what the fuss was about. If Barbara did not like housework, she should not do it. 'I won't mind,' said Tom. 'Don't do it.' Barbara took up the challenge and stopped all housework, except cooking. After the first week the kitchen was littered with dirty pans and dishes. (I remember thinking that they must have been fairly well-off to have so much crockery. In our house it's a question of having to wash up before the next meal can be prepared.) The dust piled up, and by the fourth week Barbara had to wash up pans and dishes before cooking. By the sixth week Tom was showing visible frustration and irritation, as his wife continued to spend most of her time lying comfortably in bed or on the settee, listening to music, reading her favourite novels and eating succulent grapes. 'This has gone too far,' Tom burst out. 'If you don't pull yourself together, I will call the doctor in.' When Barbara did not respond, a week later the doctor arrived and when his advice was ignored, a psychiatrist was brought in. Understandably, Barbara became very upset and cross about the whole procedure. This was interpreted as further evidence of her mental instability. In a patriarchally determined model of mental illness in which insanity is defined by the degree to which women deviate from accepted female roles and behaviour, Barbara did not stand a chance. She was taken to a psychiatric unit and was sectioned under the Mental Health Act. It is, of course, possible that this story was invented, and it could be argued that it falls outside the realms of reality. In the interest of 'research' perhaps some women would like to do what Barbara did and see what happens as a result of their deviation from expected gender roles. A psychiatric ward may not be the ultimate fate but my guess is that a chain of negative reactions, indicative of disapproval of the observed deviation, would ensue.

The focus on the general conceptualisation of women as reproducers and housewives, deviation from which merits the imposition of social control, is a useful starting point in our understanding of black women's experiences of the health service. It is also especially crucial in the British context, where black women have been subsumed into an existing framework within which female stereotypes were already well established. That conceptualisation, reflected in medical ideology, has its roots in the wider social, political and economic structure, and was epitomised by the eugenics movement.

Eugenics, which concerns selective breeding, was a strong influential movement in nineteenth-century Britain. Its aim was to create a superior white race. This was to be achieved by encouraging the middle classes, who were believed to be intelligent and responsible, to reproduce abundantly whilst the working classes, who were perceived as feckless and irresponsible, were discouraged from breeding. Some eugenicists such as Dr C. V. Drysdale, were prepared to go to the extent of withholding medical treatment to unfit working-class people who insisted on producing children. Dr Drysdale suggested that the medical profession should have two oaths, the Hippocratic, and a Darwinian one promising to save the lives of such people only if there was no possibility of their breeding:

> Success in the environment is the true test of fitness and all those who fail, either through disease, accident, or inability to gain a livelihood are the unfit whose lives may be preserved but only at the price of renouncing the right to perpetuate their type.[2]

Other eugenicists included in the category of unfit, black people, who were of course a threat to the reproduction of the superior race. Reverend James Hamilton, for example, warned against the pollution of white blood, as this would help to undermine British power and influence:

> If, for example, the policy be continued of keeping an open door for every foreigner, and especially allowing such alien and inferior breeds as negroes, Chinese and Japanese to enter, marry, and settle down in great numbers, while young people of pure British blood emigrate to other lands, this country will in a few generations have so much foreign and undesirable blood in the national veins as cannot fail to have a deleterious effect on the national character, and, as a consequence, on all those national ideals, endeavours, and achievements which we value so highly in the present day.[3]

Others thought that black people should be eliminated altogether, not just in Britain but in their own countries, in order to make room for the innately superior white race to rule. Karl Pearson, a prominent sociologist of the time, and a formidable figure behind this school of thought, wanted colonies such as South Africa to be totally dominated by this white race even if this meant genocide for the black population.[4]

During the period when the eugenicists were disseminating ideas about selective breeding, vasectomy was not a widely used form of contraception, if it was used at all, so it is reasonable to conclude that it was not men's fertility that was to be curtailed. The target group for control in this grand plan of creating a superior race was composed mainly of working-class white women with perhaps the sprinkling of black women who were living in Britain at the time. The explicit link between class, race and gender as the basis of social control and oppression was made. Any doubts about this are expelled by Marie Stopes, who today is regarded by many as the champion of working-class women. Stopes, a member of the Eugenics Society, opened the first birth control clinic for working-class women in England. Although the clinic was certainly helpful to many such women who found themselves burdened with endless, and sometimes unwanted, pregnancies through lack of contraception, Stopes stated clearly that her main concern in setting up the clinic was that without it society would allow

> the diseased, the racially negligent, the thriftless, the careless, the feeble-minded, the very lowest members of the community, to produce innumerable tens of thousands of stunned, warped and inferior infants. If they live, a large proportion of these are doomed from their very physical inheritance to be at best but only partly self-supporting, and thus to drain the resources of those classes above them which have a sense of responsibility. The better classes, freed from the cost of the institutions, hospitals, prisons and so on, principally filled by the inferior stock, would be able to afford to enlarge their own families, and at the same time not only to save human misery but to multiply a hundredfold the contribution in human life to the riches of the State.[5]

Many who may be prepared to accept the class, race and gender-based oppressive ideology embodied in eugenics may still wonder what it has to do with the social control exerted on women by the medical profession. The link becomes clear if we locate professionally some of those who were very active in the organisation. Many were prominent and influential figures within the medical profession, such as Dr C. V. Drysdale, who was quoted earlier. Dr E. W. Hope, another eugenicist, was a medical officer of health in Liverpool. Sir James Barr was president of the British Medical Association; Sir Humphrey Rolleston was physician-in-ordinary to George V.

Not only were these men powerful within their profession, they were influential in society as a whole because of their background. Their ideas on selective breeding were shared and supported by others who were similarly placed within the class structure of British society. The list includes well-known figures such as John Maynard Keynes, Sir Julian Huxley, once director-general of Unesco, and Cyril Burt. The movement, according to Clark had its female supporters as well, who included Marie Stopes, Janet Chance and Lady Frida Laski.[6] I would argue strongly that the perception held of women, particularly working-class women, as socially and sexually irresponsible, with the consequent danger that they would swamp society with undesirable offspring, was transmitted to the medical profession through this link, and formed the basis for the social control exerted on women by the profession.

In a patriarchally dominated society women are of course ascribed specific roles within the family unit, as housewives and mothers. Those with the total freedom to be mothers must also be perceived as socially and sexually responsible – a theme from the eugenics movement – hence the continuing tendency to advocate the sterilisation of some women. These stereotypes of women, long established within British society, are reinforced by the medical profession.

It was into that structure that black women were subsumed, but they came with an additional legacy. Long before their arrival in the 1950s their status had been determined by the historical processes of slavery, colonialism and imperialism. Like the rest of the black population, they were seen as the undesirable group only to be tolerated for what they could do for society. In the labour-starved economy of the 1950s black people were not only welcomed but encouraged to come to Britain, if only to work in the unattractive sectors of industry such as transport and the health service. From the 1960s onwards, however, not only has there been a concerted effort to close doors to black people through successive immigration acts, but fears have been raised about the so-called swamping of 'British culture' and the sapping of resources by black people born in Britain. Many black women have felt that some doctors see them as the target group in their attempts to reduce the black population – reminiscent of eugenic ideas.

Bryan *et al.*, reporting on their work in the black women's struggle in Britain, say:

> There are a lot of doctors who don't even bother to make a secret of the fact that they go along with the idea that we are sapping this country's resources, and see it as their professional duty to keep our numbers down. They say things like 'well, you've already got two children, so why do you need to have any more? You might as well get your tubes tied when you come in for that D & C'. It's about racism, they don't want us here anymore and they don't need our kids to work for them, so it's easier just to quietly kill us off.[7]

But there are many 'enlightened' doctors who have no tendencies towards such a form of genocide. The differential experience of health care of black and white people is seen by some in this group as a function of other factors. If black people suffer more ill-health than working-class people it is because of their culture or genetic structure, according to this explanation. Racism – which ensures that black people receive less of society's resources and which ultimately determines not only the degree of good health but also the quality of the health care they receive – is not accepted as the root of that differential experience. This form of racism cannot simply be reduced to individuals.

That is not to say there are no individual racists within the medical profession. There are many. What is argued here is that at a structural level it is the ethos and the ideologies of the profession as a whole that define and shape the health care made available to different groups. The behaviour of individuals must, of necessity, be analysed within the context of that structure, which in turn must be understood as a product of a wider social, political and economic structure, within which black women are at the sharper end of oppression.

White women suffer from sexism, and some also from class disadvantage. Black women also face these oppressions. In addition, we are seen as belonging to cultures which are defined as inferior, bizarre or pathological – that is, racism. It really does not matter much whether you are a first-, second- or third-generation Briton. If you are black you are automatically presumed to belong to a different culture. The problem with this concerns not culture as such, but the racist refusal to accept black people as having the legitimate right to equal treatment in this society. There is certainly no problem in having a different culture; many black people have and want to maintain and perpetuate their cultures. The 'problem' only arises because black culture is perceived in negative terms, to the extent that it is held responsible for the disadvantages experienced by its members. So, for example, in 1978 J. L. Patton, the medical officer of Haringey, blamed black women and their culture for the high rates of infant mortality in England:

> Five years ago, in common with the Court Report, the increasing infant mortality rate in Haringey was thought to be due to some deficiency in the community health services, but later this investigation was prompted by the idea that the nationality of the mother was relevant . . . However, on reflection, the mother's nationality could have been an indication of the life style of her immigrant group and the effect of that life style on the quality of her maternal care.

Good maternal care has helped our species to survive through centuries of war, famine and disease.[8]

The blame is put squarely on black women and their culture. It is not the health service that is inadequate. Its adequacy, argues Patton, is 'shown by the success of the native English mothers with their babies'.[9] Patton is not only reluctant to look at racism as a possible contributing factor in the observed pattern, but also shies away from class issues: he refers to the success of 'native English mothers', when it is a well-known fact that working-class children have a higher mortality rate than their middle-class counterparts.

In the area of sexuality and fertility black women have faced horrendous treatment in the health service. Maya Angelou characterises the general view that white people have of black women's sexuality: 'black women have sex but white women make love'. [10] The implication is that black women are of low moral fibre, are sex-mad and prostitutes. Some politicians, e.g., Enoch Powell and Margaret Thatcher in the 1960s and 1970s, have consistently stated their concern about the swamping of England by black people, not through immigration – that inlet has been effectively closed by parliamentary acts – but by the numbers of black people born here. This manufactured fear has played a part in the eagerness of some doctors to impose abortions and sterilisations on black women, as well as Depo Provera, a form of contraceptive, all in an attempt to reduce their fertility. This has been documented by Bryan *et al*, and is confirmed by my own experience in the health service. It is precisely for this reason that black women rejected the white feminist demand for 'the right to abortion' and instead demanded 'the right to choose' to have or not to have a baby.

However, many in the medical profession reject this view of systematic genocide. Starting from the stereotype of

27

black women as sex-mad, many health professionals believe that most, if not all, black women have had illegal abortions as a result of their promiscuousness. This assumption was made very clear to Juanita Cole, a resident of Clapham in south London.

Mrs Juanita Cole was born in Jamaica forty-eight years ago. After coming to London she developed various symptoms of ill-health and as a result she frequently visited her neighbourhood clinic, where she was quickly labelled 'the annoyance'.[11] Such an attitude had the effect of discouraging her from going, even when she started passing blood in her urine. She became frightened when, after four days, she was still passing blood. After telling a nurse about her condition, she was told that four days was not long enough to cause concern, and to come back after a week if the symptoms persisted. The nurse assured her that it was something she ate. The blood disappeared but reappeared after two months, and although the nurse told Mrs Cole over the phone not to worry, she decided to go to the clinic and this time was seen by the doctor. The doctor was interested, but more in her reproductive capacity than in her illness. He said: 'The record says you got a boy first, then two girls . . . you got a boy, then a girl, so why did you go ahead and have another one, you had one of each?' The doctor did not examine Mrs Cole. He gave her a prescription and told her to come back when she wanted. The sickness became worse and when she returned to the clinic again she was sent to the hospital, where she was examined by a consultant. On examining her, he said: 'Whoever did your abortions for you was a butcher.' When Mrs Cole told him that she had never had an abortion, his retort was: 'Mrs Cole, if you haven't had an abortion, you're the first woman of your kind who I've ever treated who hasn't.'

The specialist then turned his attention to the medical aspects of his patient: 'If you felt this way, then how come you never went to see a local doctor, someone in the clinic where you live? You must know about the health program, you've been here almost 20 years.' When Mrs Cole told him about the many visits she made to the clinic, he consulted his records and said: 'According to the information I was given, your complaints have been strictly psychological.'

Cottle, who relates Juanita Cole's experience, informs us that:

> Juanita Cole was operated on the afternoon following her admission to hospital. A radical hysterectomy was performed. Frozen tissue analysis revealed that her ovaries, fallopian tubes and cervix were filled with cancerous tissue.

Mrs Cole was aware of the seriousness of her illness. She knew from the start that when you see blood in your urine it 'can be a danger sign for cancer', hence her repeated visits to the clinic. She knew she could die and her major complaint was that it would be a wasteful death: 'Wasted because her illness could have been treated as soon as she had detected it, and wasted because it would not change the attitudes and approach of the doctors and nurses . . . there would be no lesson learned by anyone . . . and that would be the biggest waste of all.'

It is now fourteen years since Cottle reported on Mrs Cole's experience. Has the way black women and black people in general are treated in the health service changed much? A recent report, *Black Health − a Political Issue*, suggests that the situation remains the same, if not worse.[12]

What I have outlined here is the experience of black women as patients in the health service. That experience cannot be divorced from the dynamics of racism in the wider structure. It cannot be seen in isolation. As black people and as women we must work together to find ways of changing our oppression whether it occurs in health, housing, education, employment or other social and political issues. We must seek each other out in Europe and in other parts of the diaspora, and work together on common issues. We must exchange views and information on how to tackle local and national as well as international issues. Our work must meet head-on the inequality and discrimination that arise from racism, sexism and classism, in other words from black women's triple oppression. The majority of black women live not in Europe, but in the so-called 'Third World' countries. Our fight for liberation will never be achieved unless women the world over are liberated, so we must work closely with black women throughout the world. In our solidarity shall be our strength to contribute to the liberation of women and the world in general. As Sojourner Truth stated:

> If the first woman God ever made was strong enough to turn the world upside down, all alone [women, together] ought to be able to turn it back and get it right side up again.[13]

Notes

1. L. Doyal, *The Political Economy of Health*, London, Pluto, 1979.
2. Quoted in H. Clarke, *'Eugenics and Sexual Knowledge'*, PhD thesis, Liverpool University, 1988, p. 238.
3. Ibid., p. 199.
4. Ibid., p. 187.
5. Ibid., p. 240.
6. Ibid.
7. B. Bryan, S. Dadzie and S. Scafe. *The Heart of Race: Black Women's Lives in Britain*, London, Virago, 1985.
8. J. L. Patton, *Infant Death by Nationality of Mother in Borough of Haringey, 1969–1972 and 1973–1975, Public Health*, London, 1978.
9. Ibid.
10. Maya Angelou, in performance, Liverpool Philharmonic, 1991.
11. Thomas Cottle, *Black Testimony*, London, Wildwood House, 1978.
12. N. P. K. Torkington, *Black Health – a Political Issue*, Liverpool Institute of Higher Education and Catholic Association for Racial Justice, Liverpool, 1991.
13. Coretta Scott King, *Sojourner Truth*, New York, Chelsea House, 1988.

Stress and Us

....

Sheridan Burton and
Leonora Kane

> Strong enough to take the pain,
> inflicted again and again.
>   (Nina Simone)

Our interest in stress stems from our personal experiences of stress and stress-related illness. We were both born and raised in England during the 1950s, with the consequent scarcity of role models, and the struggle for a comfortable identity as Black women. One of us later spent some years with a violent, unpredictable partner (which even many years later has left discernible scars), whilst the other shared her life with an alcoholic. We have both experienced the liberation and the drawbacks of single motherhood, which we do not view from the conventional Western perspective as somehow failing. We have also both successfully undertaken higher education courses while maintaining responsibility for our children. In addition, we both still juggle home, work and social lives. We feel that these issues are not personal 'problems', but a reflection of the lives of many other Black women.

Research has shown that Black people (in Western societies) experience a disproportionately high incidence of stress-related illness. In our own cases, one of us has developed a thyroid condition and hypertension, whilst the other experiences depression and a sometimes under-active immune system. We both suffer from thrush and yeast infections, from time to time. Stress-related illness, we would argue, is a direct result of our structural position in these societies, and of the racist and sexist environment in which we live. For Black women in particular therefore, understanding and learning to deal with stress is a matter of personal survival and political necessity.

In the past ten years, stress has become a buzzword in the West. It has been promoted as a condition that pre-dominantly affects white, middle-class, male executives. More recently stress has been taken up as an issue by health educators, who have been conducting a consciousness-raising exercise among the general population, with written material aimed at particular occupational groups (teachers, nurses and social workers, to name but a few). In addition there has been much attention in the mass media, which has publicised the causes of stress and suggested strategies for living with it.

This is no accident. It is part of a broader policy shift within the National Health Service, influenced by sup-posedly relentlessly shrinking resources. This policy emphasises the individual's (as opposed to the state's) responsibility for health care.

So what does taking responsibility for our own health mean? Why is it a priority? We are advised to eat more healthily, and to take more exercise. We are advised not to indulge in activities which are detrimental to our health, such as drinking alcohol, smoking and overeating. More importance is increasingly being placed by state services on preventative health care measures – breast screening and cervical smears, for example – albeit within rigid limits and targeted towards particular groups. Breast screening is available to women in the 50-plus age group, and smears are offered on a three-yearly basis, although there is evidence of more virulent forms of cervical cancer, which become established very quickly. Obviously, both tests are offered to women on a different basis if, in the doctor's view, there is evidence of dysfunction. These measures are viewed by the authorities as part of a strategy for the maintenance of a healthy population.

This apparent philosophical shift is happening alongside the streamlining of the health service, which has undergone a drastic change in structure, funding and values. The preoccupation is with minimising the need for expensive treatments, with cost effectiveness and with the targeting of those perceived as 'most in need'. The priority seems to be to find quick solutions. Unless you have an acute illness, priority for state care is increasingly given to those whose needs are considered worthy, or who can bear the wait. God forbid that you are judged to have brought the illness on yourself, for example by being a smoker, or if you are old, fat or have a disability. The only chance of moving up the waiting list is if you can afford to pay for private health care.

At a time when the NHS is concerned with cost and with adjusting its priorities, an emphasis on stress fits in conveniently. Stress is a respectable condition, associated with the hardworking professional. It is recognised as a causal factor in a number of physical illnesses, in the incidence of mental distress and in alcohol/drug misuse, all of which are of significance to Black women. Controlling stress is preventative. It also places the main responsibility for treatment on the sufferer. Many of the strategies proposed by health educators for managing stress cost the NHS little, or are obtainable only in the complementary health field.

Diabetes mellitus, hypertension, strokes and heart disease are all major conditions associated with stress. It has been associated with less serious ailments such as cystitis, thrush and backache. Stress can also affect our speed of recovery from illness.

Stress is a necessary part of life. It provokes a natural reaction, a physiological response by our bodies, which enables us to deal with difficult situations. This reaction can be triggered by fear, anger and excitement, as well as by other emotions. Known as the 'fight or flight' response, it is the bodily defence mechanism that enabled humankind to survive and evolve. When it is triggered, the body becomes flooded with the hormone adrenalin. This increases the blood pressure and diverts oxygen-rich blood to the muscles and organs involved in fighting or running away. The problem with modern society is that we often become 'stressed out' for reasons that are more sophisticated than fear or anger, and once our bodies are awash with adrenalin we do nothing with it. Fighting or running away would work it out of the system.

Everybody experiences stress. It is not always a bad thing. It makes life more interesting, and it can be a powerful motivator. Without it, we might not achieve as much as we do. Stress becomes a problem if it is frequent or continuous, because the body does not get a chance to return to its normal non-aroused state. Chronic triggering of the fight or flight response has been shown to lead to many health problems, including an overworked endocrine system and accelerated brain cell loss. Hence the close link between stress and conditions such as diabetes mellitus and thyroid problems.

Many situations can cause a stress reaction. The demands of a job or home may cause stress/overload. Crises (and the tension and anxiety which result), can be provoked by practical problems such as unemployment or money worries, and by emotional experiences such as loss or relationship problems. Such situations may be a consequence of developmental or social change, as in the need to adapt to physical change in our bodies, or changes in status/role. Normal physical processes such as the menarche, menstruation and menopause are experienced as stressful by many women. Social attitudes towards women at these times may also be a cause of stress. Since social usefulness is seen as connected to biological function, changes in physical features or in fertility are likely to be experienced by women as negative. Premenstrual syndrome and the symptoms of menopause are now medically acknowledged conditions. Neither can we overlook the impact of pressures which stem from more general, often political concerns – being a refugee for example, and/or our often unacknowledged (and sometimes unrecognised) experiences of discrimination – pressures that are linked to the political context in which we live.

In our view, both the current literature on stress and the way that stress-related illness is managed are inadequate. We live in a society with a rigid baseline, where to be acceptable is to be white, male and heterosexual. Consequently, much of the literature and information on stress ignores any other dimension. Conventional stress management literature argues that certain times and areas of life are more likely to be stress-inducing than others. The Holmes Rahe scale,[1] reproduced below, a standard mechanism for measuring stress, identifies a number of 'stressors' and measures their impact on the individual.

Life event	Lifechange units
Death of spouse	100
Divorce	73
Separation	65
Imprisonment	63
Death of family member	63
Personal injury/illness	53
Marriage	50
Dismissal from work	47
Marital reconciliation	45
Retirement	45
Change in health of family member	44
Pregnancy	40
Sexual difficulties	39

Gain of new family member	39
Business readjustment	39
Change in financial state	38
Change in number of arguments with spouse	35
Major mortgage	32
Foreclosure of mortgage/loan	30
Change of responsibility at work	29
Son or daughter leaving home	29
Trouble with in-laws	29
Outstanding personal achievement	28
Spouse begins/stops work	26
Begin or end school	26
Change in living conditions	25
Revision of personal habits	24
Trouble with boss	23
Change in work hours/conditions	20
Change in residence	20
Change in school	20
Change in recreation	19
Change in church activities	19
Change in social activities	18
Minor mortgage or loan	17
Change in sleeping habits	16
Change in eating habits	16
Change in number of family reunions	15
Vacation	13
Christmas	12
Minor violation of the law	11

Scoring more than 300 points in one year is said to greatly increase the risk of illness. A score of 150–299 reduces the risk to 30 per cent; whilst a score of less than 150 involves a slight chance of illness. Illness is not inevitable, however. Your personality and your ability to cope largely determine how well you react.

The stressors identified on this scale are all linked to

short-term, major life events that involve changes in life-style, challenges linked to personal performance, loss, expectations that create anxiety and fear, and under-stimulation. The identified stressors make a number of assumptions. Respondents are assumed to be heterosexual, married and with a family, and sufficiently wealthy to afford their own home. Because this is the expected norm, the possibility that these assigned roles may themselves be stressors is neither acknowledged nor measured. Instead, the stressor is seen as the symptom, not the cause, as short-term rather than persistent causes of stress. The relevance of gender or of race in relation to stress is not considered.

The exclusion of this dimension also occurs in the medical arena. In our experience the clinical management of stress-related illness, like hypertension, concerns itself only with medical solutions (usually involving medication), and rarely acknowledges the social and political factors that may cause it. Despite a chronic history of hyper-tension, for example, one of us has never been asked about her personal circumstances, although the fact that she was a single parent, worked full time and is Black undoubtedly contributed to her condition. Medicine may be able to do little about the pressures we all face, but it could at least acknowledge them.

Acknowledgement of the racist and sexist context in which Black women live is crucial to an understanding of the impact of stress on us. Racism and sexism impact on us at a number of levels – personally, institutionally (both as professionals and as service users), and in our interaction with society at large. We live in a racially hostile environment, which has stereotyped views of us. The hostility takes many forms. It can be subtle. Our colleagues are 'not racist', but they expect little of us, bypass us when it comes to decision-making, and always know a better way of doing things than we do. It can be casually unconscious, blatantly antagonistic or paternalistic and condescending.

On an institutional level we confront several issues as Black people. The majority of Black women still work in low-paid jobs with little training or prospects. The main stress they are likely to experience is caused by boredom, frustration and resentment. Those who 'succeed', however, may not escape these feelings. Successful Black women are often highly qualified, especially if they are competing in a white male environment. At work we are often contained, sometimes the only token Black worker. Despite equal opportunities, we lack access to the institutional networks available to our white colleagues. In spite of a public philosophy that supports the idea of equality and opposes discrimination, achievement of real equality continues to be undermined. It is not just that we are excluded by institutional processes. We don't belong to the networks that would give us access to jobs which involve power and control over the work environment.

STRESS IN BLACK AND WHITE

Social expectations of us as Black women can be a source of stress. Pressure comes both from Black and white communities, each of which holds stereotyped ideas about us and what we should be. Common stereotypes among whites include the following: that we are strong, aggressive, sexy and available. We are said to be promiscuous and irresponsible (together with insatiable). We are assumed to be, in the main, single parents; and as parents are considered to be punitive and old-fashioned in our attitudes.

Black communities have different assumptions, although there can be overlap – we can be influenced by the mass media in the same way as white people. However, generally, Black women are assumed to be heterosexual by our own communities (no lesbians in our world!!). We are expected to be conformist. We are *good* Black women if we are mothers, are self-sacrificing, perfect homemakers, good financial managers (able to survive on a shoestring), good cooks, counsellors and supporters who are always prepared to listen and not argue.

Historically, Black women have been the key to the survival of the race. We are therefore regarded as survivors, fighters, in effect 'the heart of the race'.

To educate the man is to educate an individual. To educate the woman is to educate and liberate a nation. (Malcolm X)

There is pressure on us to maintain and promote the Black female ideal, which constantly shifts depending on the current political climate and/or conventional Black male expectations, and how we interpret them. Some current ideals range from the buppie, to the radical, to the religious, to the rude-girl/ragga/yardie. The pressure to be 'right on' whether politically, religiously or economically, can be a source of stress to women within these groups, and to those who are not interested in conforming to the stereotypes, for whatever reason. Stress is generated when we deny or belittle who we really are or what we really want to do with our lives.

Many young women are still schooled in the idea that the norm is to get married and have babies. There is enormous pressure on them to conform, and any decision to live in an alternative way, such as totally independently, is perceived as abnormal.

Our existence is denied on many levels, from the trivial to the serious. We have had to struggle in a vacuum to define our own identities. While all women are subjected to various versions of the 'ideal' body weight, size, shape and colour, Black women are measured against white norms and standards, which bear no relation to our life or reality. For example, we are denied positive and authentic reflections of ourselves in the media, and there are few successful role models – we do not get to see the spectrum of 'Black is beautiful', or our varying family patterns and abilities. The images which are advanced by the media, and informed by anthropological studies, objectify us, and have been incorporated into medical perspectives. Hence the myths that we have a lower pain threshold than white people, that life is cheap for us, that we breed like animals, that we do not need time to recover from childbirth, and that there is no point in negotiating and discussing our treatment with us, because we wouldn't understand (a privilege we share with white working-class people). Since our norms are consistently denied, this can result in a feeling of failure. There is still much ambivalence within our communities about issues such as 'good' hair/'bad' hair, natural vs. processed hair (or wigs), and fair skin/dark skin. Self–image (for Black women) is closely associated with personal validation and recognition by ourselves and our communities, in a way that it isn't for white women, who are validated through their networks. We cannot rely on society in the same way. As the song says:

> If you're white, you're alright,
> If you're brown, stick around,
> If you're Black, get back.

> From 'Black, Brown and White Blues',
> Big Bill Broonzy

We have had to struggle politically to develop an identity – to be Black and proud. This means that the way we present ourselves can be seen as a form of political statement.

Black women's lives are stressful. The source of this is woven into the fabric of our existence. Sometimes the greatest stresses come from within, and are linked with the conflict between our expectations of ourselves, and reality. Many of us put everybody in the universe before ourselves and our needs. We must recognise our own importance.

Making our own space should be a priority. This is not selfish. One source of stress is about doing too much, and we need to learn to manage our time more realistically. This is likely to mean that we become more positive about ourselves and our achievements, as well as that we are more successful in what we do choose to undertake.

The key to managing stress lies in identifying what works for you, and being comfortable with the identity you have created for yourself. You may find that this takes the form of exercise, whether it is a swim, a walk, aerobics, weights, good sex, or even a vigorous bout of housework. Learning to relax is also important. So many of us juggle so much and forget how to sit down and 'chill out'. A long bath, listening to music, watching a video, having a drink to unwind, and talking to friends are some ways of doing this.

Complementary therapies are excellent – between us we have experienced aromatherapy, reflexology, acupuncture, homeopathy and Bach flower remedies. It is always worth getting a recommendation, and many therapists operate a sliding scale of fees to ensure that they are accessible to people.

We need to recognise how to identify and express our feelings. For example, very often we hold our anger in. Conversely, we often don't congratulate ourselves on our successes. We must also relearn how to share our feelings with each other. This is not a sign of weakness, but the traditional African way of life. Yes, this may make us feel vulnerable, but sharing with trusted friends and relatives is liberating, inasmuch as it reassures us that our situation and feelings are not unique, and that others have already experienced them.

Most importantly, we need to be aware that being Black and being a woman attracts pressure. For us it has been important to understand and recognise the sources of stress, and its impact on our minds and bodies. Understanding is a step towards taking control of our lives.

We are not entirely negative about the official recognition of stress, but would argue that institutions need to take on board the issues, and look at creative ways of integrating appropriate management strategies into their practice.

Note

1. Karsta, A. *The Book of Stress Survival*, Gaia Books Ltd, London, 1986.

Black Women and Hypertension

Jenny Douglas

My aim here is to review available information in present literature on black women and hypertension, to report upon current practice in medical/nursing arenas for screening for and treating hypertension and finally, and perhaps of most importance, to look at ways in which we (black women) can mobilise to prevent the high incidence of hypertension in our communities. It is important to stress that for the purpose of this chapter the review will be restricted to examining hypertension in African-Caribbean communities in the UK.

BLOOD PRESSURE

Blood pressure is represented by two numbers, for example 120/80. The top number refers to the systolic blood pressure and is the pressure exerted on the walls of the blood vessels when blood is pumped out of the heart into the arteries. The diastolic pressure is the lower number and is the pressure of blood remaining in the blood vessels when the heart relaxes. Normal blood pressure is dependent upon the physical condition of a person and blood pressure below 140/90 is thought to be normal (140 is the systolic pressure and 90 is the diastolic pressure). Anything outside the range 100–140 (systolic) and 60–90 (diastolic) is abnormal.

HYPERTENSION

Hypertension can be defined as persistently raised blood pressure. It is a silent disease, as many people can have hypertension without any symptoms or indeed without feeling unwell. There is no precise definition of hypertension as there is no clearcut dividing line between hypertension and normal blood pressure. Blood pressure varies according to a number of factors.

The exact cause of high blood pressure is not known but many factors including gender, age, diet, genetic inheritance and socioeconomic circumstances as well as psychological and emotional factors are thought to affect blood pressure. A substantial number of people are born with a tendency towards high blood pressure. This could be a true hereditary tendency, but may also be due to an individual's lifestyle and circumstances, which may be the same as those of their parents and could therefore account for increased blood pressure.

Blood pressure goes up with age. Blood pressure in children is lower than in adults, rises with age and stabilises in adulthood. Blood pressure is also associated with obesity. In the Framingham Study (1980) in the USA patients who were 10 per cent or more over their ideal weight were eight times more likely to become hypertensive than those who maintained ideal weight.

Lifestyle also plays its part – high-fat, high-sugar, high-salt diets cause obesity, which is also a risk factor for hypertension. African–Caribbean diets can be very healthy, but they can also be high in fat, sugar and salt. The high intake of salt in Caribbean diets may be of importance, particularly the ratio of sodium to potassium.

Although the stress of migration from the Caribbean to the UK and migration from rural to urban areas has been suggested as a possible factor in explaining increased blood pressure, research in Jamaica has demonstrated greater mean systolic blood pressure in agricultural workers in rural areas compared with city workers. Complex sociocultural factors including stress are responsible for other social class differences that have been reported; higher social class was associated with higher blood pressure in males while lower social class was associated with higher blood pressure in females.

DIABETES

Hypertension is also related to diabetes. There an increased prevalence of casual hypertension (hypertension on a first screening) in black diabetics when compared with white diabetics (Cruickshank and Alleyne, 1981). It is possible that hypertension could be an important primary risk factor for outcome in diabetes treatment, but there is little research in this area. There is also limited research into diabetes mellitus in the African-Caribbean communities in the UK, so the exact prevalence of the condition is as yet unknown. Research undertaken in a hospital clinic population (Nikolaides et al., 1981) and in a particular community (Odughesan et al., 1989) suggests that the prevalence of diabetes is higher in African-Caribbean communities: 2.2 per cent when compared with 1.0–1.2 per cent in the white British population. There is insufficient research to determine whether the incidence of diabetes is higher in the migrant African-Caribbean community in the UK when compared to indigenous populations in the Caribbean. The main age group for increased levels of diabetes is 45 to 64 in African-Caribbean communities, which is similar to that for Asians and whites in the UK. The frequency of insulin-dependent diabetes is thought to be lower than in white populations (Odughesan et al., 1989). Obesity is a known risk factor for both hypertension and diabetes.

Diabetes is also prevalent in older African-Caribbean populations in the Caribbean. In diabetic patients who are over 60 years 53 per cent are likely to have hypertension and 45 per cent to suffer from obesity. Diabetes is a related factor in 7 per cent of all deaths in the Caribbean.

WHY BLACK WOMEN AND HYPERTENSION?

Hypertension is more prevalent in African-Caribbean communities, particularly in women. The reasons for this are unclear. It is known that African–Caribbean women are more likely to have a genetic predisposition. However, experiences of migration from the Caribbean to the UK and the ensuing experience of racial discrimination and dis-advantage which has shaped and determined black people's socioeconomic position, are also factors. Black women are more likely to experience poverty and stress, which may add to any underlying genetic predisposition.

Many black women in Britain experience a number of types of oppression including racism, sexism and poverty. Black women are more likely to live in poor housing, have poorly paid jobs, work part-time, work outside the home while bringing up a family, be caring for other relatives and be exposed to occupational health hazards because of the nature of their work. Black women are also more likely to work nights and long shifts. Research, particularly on black women working in health services, demonstrates that black women experience both racism and sexism at work and because of this are less likely to hold positions that are commensurate with their skills, experience and training. Thus many black women experience stress associated with work. The financial responsibility of many black households falls on black women because racism and discrimination experienced by black men results in larger numbers being unemployed as compared to their white counterparts.

Because of their socioeconomic and environmental circumstances, black women are also more likely to suffer from particular types of disease and ill-health. Cerebro-vascular disease, hypertension and strokes are some of the conditions more common in African-Caribbean women.

COMPARATIVE DATA FOR HYPERTENSION/ STROKE

It is important to look at comparisons between ethnic groups for differences in blood pressure, hypertension and stroke in order to determine possible reasons for the reported differences. Research shows that hypertension and cerebrovascular disease are more common among British people of African and African-Caribbean origin than among other ethnic groups. Hypertension has long been recognised as a major black health problem in the USA. However there is little research which compares the prevalence of hypertension in the African-Caribbean population in the UK with African-Caribbean populations in the Caribbean. Thus we have no knowledge of how the experience of migration itself has affected the health status of African-Caribbean communities in the UK.

In the previous section I reported that both genetic and environmental factors determine levels of blood pressure. I will now try to bring together existing research findings in the UK, the USA and the Caribbean in order to try and compare experiences of hypertension and stroke in African-Caribbean populations.

In population studies it has been demonstrated that high blood pressure tends to run in families. Studies have also revealed marked differences between 'racial' groups, although it has not been possible to determine whether the differences are due to environmental or genetic influences. Studies in the USA have shown that in the USA more black people have high blood pressure than white people. Prevalence in black people is reported to be up to four times that observed in white people, with severe elevations (diastolic blood pressure above 115 mmHg) being five to seven times more common (Report of the Secretary's Task Force on Black and Minority Health, 1986). Black people also have a higher death rate – three times higher from hypertension when compared to whites (Gillum, 1982; Gillum and Grant 1982). Black people also develop the disease at a younger age, and the severity of the disease is greater. Black women have lower blood pressure in early adult life than black men. By the age of 50 both the systolic and diastolic pressures of the women catch up with those of men. The same gender differences can be found in young white adults but women catch up with men at a later age than is the case for black people – in their 60s and 70s.

In the UK diastolic blood pressure of 130 mmHg or more is found in about 0.5 per cent of the total population. There are insufficient studies of blood pressure levels in black populations in Britain, but from the studies that do exist average blood pressure among black populations in the Caribbean, West Africa and Britain do not appear to be substantially different to those of whites. This is contrary to the findings in the USA, where blood pressure is found to be consistently higher in black populations.

An examination of mortality rates for hypertension and cerebrovascular disease between 1970 and 1972 in different ethnic groups showed that people born in Africa had 4.5 times, and people born in the Caribbean up to 6.6 times, the mortality rate of people born in England and Wales (Marmot et al., 1981). When the figures for mortality from stroke were compared for the years 1979–83 there were 76 per cent more deaths for men born in the Caribbean and 110 per cent more for women born in the Caribbean when compared with rates for England and Wales as a whole (Balarajan, 1991).

African-Caribbeans have lower rates of coronary heart disease than white and Asian communities; however the research demonstrates that deaths from stroke in Britain are highest in African-Caribbean communities. Hence, rather than suggesting that hypertension is no more of a problem for black than for white communities, the mortality differences do highlight that perhaps more research on blood pressure levels in black populations in Britain is required, as it also appears that African and African-Caribbean people are more likely to suffer a stroke than white people at a given level of blood pressure (Stamler *et al.*, 1974).

EFFECTS OF HYPERTENSION

Hypertension is usually without any symptoms, and individuals may feel quite well until complications develop. Reported symptoms then include headache, dizziness, stroke, dyspnoea, ankle swelling and chest pains, visual problems and heart attack.

Raised blood pressure is one of the conventional risk factors for coronary heart disease along with smoking, high serum cholesterol, hypothyroidism, stress, reduced exercise, and increased consumption of alcohol. Although ischaemic heart disease (heart attack) is less common in African-Caribbeans than in whites, the most common clinical complications of hypertension in African-Caribbeans are stroke, renal failure, congestive cardiac failure, enlarged heart, and impairment or loss of vision. Hypertension shortens life by damaging target organs, especially the heart, brain and kidneys.

Heart
In individuals with hypertension, the heart is forced to pump blood against increased resistance for many years, which leads to enlargement of the heart and eventually to heart failure and death. Coronary heart disease is more common in people with hypertension.

The brain

Stroke is caused by interruption of the blood supply to the brain and is the most common consequence of hypertensive damage to the brain. Hypertension is the single most important cause of strokes in African-Caribbeans.

The kidneys

Hypertension directly affects the kidneys, causing renal damage and eventually renal failure. Kidney damage itself can cause high blood pressure, which in turn may cause further kidney damage.

Untreated hypertension sets up a vicious cycle of events. Elevated blood pressure will continue to rise even further if left untreated and in addition to the effects already outlined on target organs, impairment or loss of vision can occur.

Pregnancy and oral contraception

High blood pressure can occur in pregnancy or while taking oral contraception. Pregnancy-induced hypertension includes clinical conditions of hypertension, oedema (generalised swelling, particularly of the hands and feet) and proteinuria (traces of protein in the urine). Pre-eclampsia and eclampsia are two categories of pregnancy-induced hypertension. Pre-eclampsia is hypertension with proteinuria and/or oedema after the twentieth week of gestation. Eclampsia is an extension of the pre-eclamptic stage, and characterised by seizures.

Pregnancy-induced hypertension occurs in about 5–7 per cent of all pregnancies, but is higher in low-income patients and in groups where chronic hypertension is high (for example black women). The risk of pregnancy-induced hypertension in high-risk groups is five times higher than for women with normal blood pressure. In the

UK, pregnancy-induced hypertension is the leading cause of maternal death. Some studies of African-Caribbean women in the Caribbean have demonstrated that women who had not had children seemed to be at greater risk of hyper-tension than those who had had children. When compared with women with normal pregnancies, those women who had had pre-eclamptic toxaemia showed a greatly increased prevalence of hypertension. Twenty six per cent of all maternal deaths in a study in Jamaica were shown to be related to hypertensive disease (Grell, 1989). It has long been recognised that oral contraceptives produce an elevation in blood pressure. The combined pill should not be used by women with chronic hypertension, although some clinicians consider that the mini-pill is safe for use, depending upon the severity of hypertension.

DIAGNOSIS AND TREATMENT

The diagnosis and treatment of hypertension varies from country to country. In the USA epidemiological data has shown that benefits can be derived from treating both black and white hypertensive patients' diastolic blood pressures above 90 mmHg. In the Caribbean a practical working diagnosis is a repeated blood pressure level above 160/10 mmHg. In the UK blood pressure is treated at diastolic pressures of 100mmHg or more. In patients under 65 years treatment would be aimed at keeping the pressure below 140/90 mmHg.

There is also divergence in the drugs normally used to lower blood pressure in the UK and in the Caribbean. Research suggests that there may be differences in the way that hypertensive patients of different ethnic groups respond to the various drugs commonly used to lower blood pressure (Mares et al., 1985). This means that specific drugs may be more or less efficacious or toxic in different ethnic groups and may produce different or more severe side-effects.

There is a range of anti-hypertensive drugs, including betablockers and diuretics, and drugs may be given in different combinations. Mounting evidence now suggests that particular drugs or combinations of drugs should be used in African-Caribbean patients. Some medication causes side-effects such as dizziness, depression, tiredness, and impotence in men. One of the reasons some people cease their medication is that they start to feel unwell because of side-effects. It is important for such patients to discuss this with their GP so that they can be prescribed a more suitable drug.

SERVICE PROVISION

There is still no consensus among doctors about when high blood pressure becomes hypertension and at what point treatment should start. The definition of hypertension used by the World Health Organisation is 160/95 mmHg. Torkington (1991) in a study conducted in Liverpool, reported that there was great variation in physicians' attitudes and definitions, but that overall they would recommend treatment with a rise in diastolic pressure in relation to age:

91–95   in the 30–49 age group
101–105   in the 50–69 age group
110+   in the over 70s age group

There is also divergence on whether or not treatment is beneficial to all patients who have elevated blood pressure.

Bannan, Beevers and Wright (1981) report that about 0.5 per cent of the middle-aged population have diastolic blood pressure of 130 mmHg or more; a further 4 per cent have diastolic pressures of 110–29 mmHg and about 20 per cent of such people will die in five years if left untreated. People with diastolic pressures of 90 mmHg have a shorter life expectancy and those with pressures below 90, for example a 35-year-old man with a diastolic pressure of 100 mmHg, can expect a sixteen-year reduction in life expectancy. For people with mild hypertension there is a greater risk of heart attack and stroke, so early screening and detection are particularly important.

SCREENING

General practitioners should ensure that adequate and appropriate screening facilities are available and accessible to all sections of the population. Present research demonstrates that women, especially black women and working-class women, experience worse treatment from health services (Douglas, 1992). This is of particular concern in relation to primary health services where, when black women present with illness, physical symptoms may be interpreted as psychological or psychosomatic and hypertension may not be detected until damage to some organs has occurred and when it is too late for non-drug therapy to be implemented. It is also possible that for some black women, general practitioners are too keen to implement a regime of drug therapy without having explored intervention such as dietary modification, exercise and stress management. Little health education and health promotion information is targeted at African-Caribbean communities. More information needs to be produced and made available to black women.

Screening facilities should be established in community centres, churches and recreation centres so that people who do not visit general practitioners are not missed. Early detection and treatment can reduce mortality from strokes and heart attacks.

PREVENTING HYPERTENSION

Although there is conflicting evidence about the benefit of treating hypertension, all the evidence suggests that emphasis should initially be placed on prevention and non-drug therapies. Healthy lifestyles may prevent hypertension in black women or at least delay it, in spite of the hereditary trend. Attention to weight gain, maintaining a healthy diet, being physically active, avoiding excessive amounts of alcohol and not smoking cigarettes are all ways in which we can reduce the risk of hypertension.

In addition studies have shown that a high-fibre, high-potassium diet lowers blood pressure. Vegetables and fruits are excellent sources of fibre and potassium. Research has also demonstrated that vegetarian diets have been associated with lowering blood pressure and although the exact mechanism is not clear, it may be due to the combined effect of high fibre and high potassium with low fat and low sodium in such diets.

In individuals with mild hypertension, diet could play an important role in managing and reducing blood pressure. Obesity is the single condition most often associated with hypertension. A healthy diet is important for weight reduction. The traditional Caribbean diet is healthy (Douglas, 1987, 1989) but changes have occurred in this as a result of migration, socioeconomic circumstances, food advertising and food availability. It is important that information on healthy eating should be relevant and appropriate to African-Caribbean communities.

There are very strong, widely held beliefs about food and health in African-Caribbean communities, some of them based on traditional beliefs. Many people believe that the white variety of the vegetable cho-cho (christophene) relieves high blood pressure. Purgatives made of herbs are popular and are also thought to relieve high blood pressure. Many herbal or 'bush teas' used throughout the Caribbean are derived from the African heritage and tradition of the use of herbal medicines. Most bush teas are useful, and the drinking of herbal teas is undoubtedly preferable to tea or coffee containing caffeine, which is known to elevate blood pressure. However, problems can arise when people attempt to cure hypertension only by the use of bush teas and reduce or discard medically prescribed medication, with damaging results.

Grell (1985) suggests that mild hypertension (diastolic blood pressure between 90 and 104 mmHg and where there are no coronary risk factors and no target organ damage) can be controlled by the following.

Reducing salt in the diet

Food may be cooked or canned with salt, but no salt should be added after cooking. Salt used in preparation of food should be limited to one teaspoon daily. Food with a high sodium content (for example ham, bacon, sausage, salted fish or meat, crisps, salted crackers) should be omitted. Spices should be used for flavour instead of salt.

Reducing weight

Obesity may cause problems in addition to hypertension such as diabetes and coronary heart disease. The following guidelines should be borne in mind to manage obesity: eat meals at specific times; eat moderate amounts of food at each meal; eat only until just satisfied and do not overeat; don't skip meals; eat some foods high in fibre – corn, wholewheat flour, rice, breadfruit, yams, plantain, banana, pulses, nuts, vegetables and fruit; avoid snacking or eating because bored, depressed or upset; eat fewer fats, sugars and starchy foods.

Reducing intake of dietary fat

Vegetable-oil-based margarine and cooking oil (not coconut oil or red palm oil) substituted for butter and animal products have been shown to lower blood pressure in hypertensive patients. Using high polyunsaturated and low saturated fats also reduces the risk of coronary artery disease in hypertensives by lowering total cholesterol and low-density proteins by 10–15 per cent.

Reducing alcohol in the diet

A reduction of alcohol to less than two or three drinks a day in heavy drinkers who are hypertensive has been shown to reduce blood pressure.

Reducing smoking

Cigarette smoking is a major risk factor for coronary artery disease and there is an association between cigarette smoking and renovascular hypertension.

Non-dietary management

This includes exercise, relaxation (stress reduction), meditation and yoga.

Blood pressure should be checked frequently, and individuals should be aware of what their blood pressure is and what it means. We should not assume that our blood pressure is normal if we feel well, as the early stages of hypertension are symptom free.

Earlier I outlined the research on hypertension and pregnancy. It is particularly important that black women receive appropriate antenatal care and that service providers ensure that it is relevant and accessible to African-Caribbean women. Similarly, attention must be focused on appropriate screening and counselling for African-Caribbean women in contraception services to ensure that contraceptives which increase blood pressure are not prescribed.

We must not lose sight of the fact that increasingly research in the UK is highlighting the association between socioeconomic circumstances and coronary heart disease and stress (Marmot, 1988). Although there is growing research linking the high incidence of coronary heart disease in black Americans with disadvantage and poor economic status, little research in the UK has examined the role played by poverty, racism and stress on blood pressure in African-Caribbean communities. More research on the prevalence of hypertension and the average blood pressure in African-Caribbean communities in the UK is required to ensure that appropriate screening and treatment procedures are developed and adopted.

Many factors are known to increase stress — including unemployment, poor living conditions, poverty and isolation. For many black people in Britain the experience of racism increases stress and may be one of a number of factors causing hypertension. Poverty and stress may be difficult to address on an individual basis. However, it is important to articulate our needs and experiences in order to ensure that services and the basic needs we all have for housing, education and good health are met in a just and fair manner. For most black women this means fighting the many oppressions we face in this society.

COMMUNITIES ORGANISING
Black women's groups, churches and community groups should organise to ensure that information about high blood pressure and other health concerns is widely available to everyone.

Information on healthy eating and the reduction of stress

can be disseminated widely. Self-help groups, organised around increasing physical activities, reducing smoking and reducing stress, can be of great benefit to people with mild hypertension. Knowledge of the importance of regular blood pressure checks and of being aware of your blood pressure can be disseminated through community groups and networks. Such community organisations can press for more adequate research on the levels of blood pressure in black communities in the UK and research on appropriate treatment methods. Better information and service provision could greatly reduce deaths in black communities.

There is a need for more research on the incidence and prevalence of hypertension in African–Caribbean communities in the UK. More investigation into the nature of diabetes and hypertension is also needed, and the implications of the results of this research for treatment of both conditions. The effects of drug therapy on hypertension in different ethnic groups also warrants further research. Indeed, we need more research that focuses on the links between hypertension and stress and the specific implications of this for black women. Finally, black women need to be more centrally involved in setting the research agenda and in developing strategies for health education and promotion in our communities.

References

Adams, L., Watkins, L., Kuller, L., Savage, B., Donahue, R. & LaPorte, R. (1986) 'The Relationship of Social Class to Coronary Heart Disease Risk Factors in Blacks: The Implications of Social Mobility or Risk Factor Change,' Report of the Secretary's Task Force on Black and Minority Health, US Department of Health & Human Services, US, Government Printing Office, Washington, DC, p. 285–99.

Balarajan, R. (1991) 'Ethnic Differences in Mortality from Ischaemic Heart Disease and Cerebrovascular Disease in England and Wales', *British Medical Journal*, 302: 560–4.

Bannan, L. T., Beevers, D. G. and Wright, N. (1981) 'The Size of the Problem' in *ABC of Hypertension*, *British Medical Journal*, 1981, pp. 18–20.

Cruikshank, J. K. and Alleyne, S. A. (1981) 'Vascular Disease in West Indian and White Diabetics in Britain and Jamaica', *Postgraduate Medical Journal*, December, 1981, Vol. 57, pp. 766–8.

Cruickshank, J. K. and Alleyne, S. A. (1987) 'Black West Indian and Matched White Diabetics in Britain compared with Diabetics in Jamaica: BM, BP and Vascular Disease', *Diabetes Care*, 10 (2): 170–9.

Cruickshank, J. K. and Beevers, D. G. (1989) *Ethnic Factors in Health and Disease*, Kent, Wright.

Cruickshank, J. K., Beevers, D. G., Osbourne, V. L., Haynes, R. A., Corlett, J. C. R. and Selby, S., (1980) 'Heart Attack, Stroke, Diabetes and Hypertension in West Indians, Asians and Whites in Birmingham, England', *British Medical Journal*, 2: 1108–9.

Douglas, J. (1987) *Caribbean Food and Diet*, 'Training in Health and Race', National Extension College, Cambridge.

Douglas, J. (1989) 'Food Type Preferences and Trends among Afro-Caribbeans in Britain', in J. Cruickshank and D. G. Beevers (eds), *Ethnic Factors in Health and Disease*, Kent, Wright.

Douglas, J. (1992) 'Black Women's Health Matters', in H. Roberts (ed.), *Women's Health Matters*, London, Routledge.

Gillum, R. F. (1982) 'Coronary Heart Disease in Black Populations. I: Mortality and Morbidity', *American Heart Journal*, 104: 839.

Gillum, R. F. and Grant, C. T. (1982) 'Coronary Heart Disease in Black Populations. II: Risk Factors', *American Heart Journal* 104: 852.

Grell, G. A. C. (1983) 'Hypertension in the West Indies', *Postgraduate Medical Journal*, 59: 616–21.

Grell, G. A. C. (1985), 'Hypertension Control in the Caribbean', *Cajanus* Vol. 18, No. 3, pp. 131–9.

Grell, G. A. (1989) 'Management of Hypertension in the Caribbean: the Jamaican Perspective', in J. Cruickshank and D. G. Beevers (eds), *Ethnic Factors in Health and Disease*, Kent, Wright.

Haynes, S., Feinleib, M., and Kannel, W. (1980) 'The Relationship of Psychosocial Factors to Coronary Heart Disease: The Framington Study 3–8-Year Incidence of Coronary Heart Disease', *American Journal of Epidemiology*, Vol. 3, No. 37.

James, S. (1984) 'Socioeconomic Influences on Coronary Heart Disease in Black Populations', *American Heart Journal* 108: 669.

Kasl, S. V. (1984) 'Social and Psychologic Factors in the Etiology of Coronary Heart Disease in Black Populations: An Exploration of Research Needs', *American Heart Journal* 108: 660.

Mares, P., Henley, A. and Baxter, C. (1985) *Health Care in Multiracial Britain*, Cambridge, Health Education Council/National Extension College.

Marmot, M. G. (1988) 'Psychosocial factors and Cardiovascular Disease: Epidemiological Approaches', *European Heart Journal*, pp. 690–7.

Marmot, M. G., Adelstein, A. M. and Bulusu, L. (1981) 'Cardiovascular Mortality among Immigrants to England and Wales', *Postgraduate Medical Journal*, December. 57: 760–2.

Nikolaides, K., Barnett, A. H., Spirolopoulos, A. J. and Watkins, P. J. (1981) 'West Indian Diabetic Population of a Large Inner City Diabetic Clinic', *British Medical Journal*, 283: 1374–5.

Odughesan, O., Rone, B., Fletcher, J. (1989) 'Diabetes in the UK West Indian Community: the Wolverhampton Survey', *Diabetic Medicine*, 6: 48–52.

Stamler, J., Schoenberger, J. A., Shekelle, R. D., and Stamler, R. (1974) 'Hypertension: The Problem and the Challenge', in *The Hypertension Handbook*, Merck, Sharp and Dohme, Westpoint, Pennsylvania.

Torkington, N. P. K. (1991) *Black Health – A Political Issue*, Liverpool, Catholic Association for Racial Justice and Liverpool Institute of Higher Education.

White, E. (ed.) (1990) *The Black Women's Health Book*, Seattle, Washington, Seal Press.

Women and Sickle Cell Disorders

Elizabeth N. Anionwu

> I'm 31 now, and I didn't expect to make it to this age.
> I believe I'll die earlier than most women do, and I'm still in
> a big rush to live life as fully as possible in the time I have.
> I feel I could have made it a long time ago – in my singing
> and my designing – if my health had been normal, because
> I have got the determination to succeed. Sickle cell has
> caused me a lot of grief. But it's also taught me to be strong
> and positive. (Margaret Deacon, 1991)

Personal accounts about the effects of sickle cell anaemia,
such as the above by Margaret, who was featured in
Woman's Own magazine, have started to increase awareness
of the impact of this chronic inherited blood disorder.
The grief that Margaret refers to is in part due to the
unpredictable and variable nature of the illness. At times it
is possible to think (incorrectly) that the illness is no longer
present, after years without problems. Then it can strike
without warning and disrupt normal routines with
excruciating pains, severe infections, anaemia and damage
to various parts of the body.

Here I will focus on the effects on women of one type
of sickle cell disorder – sickle cell anaemia – the most
common and usually the most severe type. Similar problems
can occur in the other types such as haemoglobin SC

disease and sickle thalassaemia, but may be less severe and less frequent, although this is not always the case. The problems that can occur from childhood into adulthood will be described using excerpts from Margaret's story to illustrate various themes.

A CHILD WITH SICKLE CELL ANAEMIA

A child born with sickle cell anaemia has inherited it from both parents – it is not an illness that can be caught like chickenpox. It affects boys and girls in equal numbers. The parents of a child with sickle cell anaemia are probably healthy carriers of *sickle cell trait*, found in about one in ten Afro-Caribbeans and one in four West Africans. It is also found in other ethnic groups such as Mediterraneans, Asians and people from the Middle East. Sickle cell trait, but not sickle cell anaemia, appears to offer some protection from malaria in early childhood. If both parents have sickle cell trait every child they have could inherit sickle cell anaemia, sickle cell trait or nothing at all. This means that all, none or some of their children could be affected.

TESTING

Sickle cell trait and sickle cell anaemia are detected through a special blood test that can be arranged by family doctors, or at the sickle cell centres that now exist in approximately twenty-four health authorities in England and Wales (Anionwu, in press).

SICKLE CELL ANAEMIA IN CHILDHOOD

I was always a poorly child – forever weak and out of breath, with chest and arm pains. . . . Sickle cell weakens the body's immunity to illness, so I suffered far more than my share of childhood ailments. I remember when I was about 12 I became very sick with pneumonia and ended up having to go into hospital. Several doctors stood around my bed – I was pretending to be asleep because I hate crowds – and one said, 'This young lady has sickle cell anaemia.' That was the first time that I'd heard of it. I didn't know what it meant and I didn't really want to know. My parents hadn't heard of sickle cell either.

Lack of awareness about sickle cell anaemia in our community and amongst health professionals was a key factor in my involvement with setting up, in Brent in 1979, the first sickle cell information, screening and counselling centre in Britain. Research that I undertook in 1981 with twenty-two parents (mainly mothers) revealed that only one had ever heard of the condition before her child was diagnosed with the illness (Anionwu, 1988). This is not surprising, in view of the lack of information in the media, schools and in the training of health professionals. For example, I trained as a nurse in Paddington in the late 1960s and never had a lecture on the condition. This was a fairly universal observation and was confirmed in my research, which included a study conducted in 1980, amongst 154 health visitors and school nurses in London.

SICKLING

The problems associated with sickle cell anaemia usually do not occur until after the age of four to six months, even though the illness can be detected in the unborn and newborn baby. After this age the red blood cells can change from a doughnut shape to that resembling a banana, half-moon or a farmer's sickle. This tends to occur if the body has a lowered level of oxygen or fluid. Factors that can bring on sickling include infection and fever, strenuous exercise, sudden change of temperature, consumption of alcohol, pregnancy and stress.

These odd 'sickle'-shaped red blood cells block small blood vessels, particularly in the bones. They can cause mild to excruciating pain – 'the painful crisis' – which accounts for up to 90 per cent of hospital admissions of patients with sickle cell anaemia. Sickling in the spleen can give rise to sudden anaemia and swelling of the abdomen, and is life-threatening. A less common but very severe complication of sickle cell anaemia in childhood is stroke, caused by blockage of the blood vessels in the brain. Other problems can include bedwetting until late adolescence, yellowness in the whites of the eyes and delay in puberty, such as delay in growth and late onset of periods. Children with sickle cell anaemia may have a poor appetite and be thin, although this is not always the case.

Affected individuals may have several hospital admissions a year. Some may rarely be affected, whereas others may be constantly in hospital, causing disruption to schooling, employment and family life:

> I felt isolated throughout my school days. I was often absent because of illness, so never had the chance to make real friends. In my teens I was a real bore. I couldn't enjoy games because the cold affected me so badly, making my limbs ache. It was so painful. The teachers thought that I just wanted to get out of games, but I really did feel ill. They couldn't see that I was telling the truth, and I'd never admit I had sickle cell. I'd say, 'My arm aches', or, 'My leg aches', and the teacher would dismiss me saying, 'Yes, Margaret, now go out on to the field.' So I used to participate, in the cold, aching and miserable, but still I couldn't talk to anyone about it.

The above quote from Margaret highlights the stigma and isolation that a young person can experience with a chronic illness such as sickle cell anaemia. In addition it is an illness that is of particular significance for black and minority ethnic populations, with resulting effects of racism and marginalisation. However, it is important to stress that it does also occur in whites, for example Greeks.

TREATMENT OF SICKLE CELL ANAEMIA

Affected individuals are advised to:

drink plenty of fluids;

take a small dose of penicillin every day to avoid the risk of certain infections (particularly in childhood and adolescence);

be fully immunised and take anti-malarial precautions in the tropics;

avoid extremes of temperatures;

have a well-balanced diet;

have sufficient rest and avoid over-exertion;

receive prompt medical attention if they have a fever, become very tired and pale, have a swollen abdomen, become chesty, develop weakness down one side of the body and if the painful crisis is not controlled by care and medication at home. In respect to children, the mother is usually the carer and should be encouraged to have confidence in her own knowledge and suspicions, and seek medical advice when she has a gut feeling that her child is not well.

Sharon Edwards had sickle cell anaemia. She died in November 1992, as a result of the disease. Before her death, at the age of 30, she wrote about her personal feelings of having the disease, including its effects on her childhood. In the following account, from 'A Personal View of Sickle Cell Pain', she describes how she learned she had the disease.

I am 29 years old, and was born with sickle cell disease but I wasn't diagnosed until I was 5 years old. Until the age of 5 I was treated for rheumatism. When I was 5 I had a lot of pain in my side and I was rushed to hospital and diagnosed as having appendicitis. I was prepared for theatre, my parents signed the consent form, and just as I was about to actually go into theatre the Sister said, let's do a sickle cell test first.

They did and found that I was HbSS [sickle cell anaemic] and then they diagnosed it was not my appendix. My parents were tested and found to be carriers, yet they didn't know what sickle cell was and had never heard of it. My two brothers both have the trait as well. My Mum's Mum died when my Mum was 3 years old and looking back, she was always in pain and unwell; they think that she had sickle cell disease too and it had come down in the family.

Growing up as a child I used to be very, very sick. I used to have crises at school every week or two. I missed a lot of school and my education was badly affected. When I was 10 years old my parents were told that I wouldn't live to be 13 because I was so ill. I was having transfusions every four to six weeks for three years at one stage.

(Sharon Edwards, 1993)

Medical treatment will include pain relief for home use as well as very strong drugs during hospital admission (e.g. pethidine or diamorphine). During hospital admissions the patient may receive fluids into the veins to avoid dehydration. Blood transfusions may be used during times of sudden and life-threatening complications. Occasionally they may be used every month, following a stroke, or if a patient has been severely and frequently incapacitated because of painful crises. They may also be given during pregnancy. However, blood transfusions carry a risk of reactions or infections, and may leave too much iron in the body. Therefore they are not a routine part of treatment in sickle cell anaemia. Sharon Edwards describes the result of one side-effect – too much iron:

About 3 to 4 years ago I had a liver infection and the doctor told me I had iron overload. I didn't know what she was talking about, and I understand that the normal level for iron in your blood should be less than 300µg/1. When they diagnosed I had an iron overload it was 8000µg/1. She told me I had to use a Desferal pump. She took me into a room, showed me slides, and explained to me that I would have to use this pump maybe for life, or for a few years until my iron level does come down. At one stage I said, 'No, I can't deal with this, because it has been one thing after another. I don't want this, I can't do it, I can't inject myself and I don't want it.' She said, 'Sharon, if you don't take it, within a couple of years you will be dead, because the iron is so high it will affect your liver, your heart and your kidneys.' So I went away and thought about it and I started using it.

Affected individuals are living into adulthood and some are now surviving into their 50s and 60s. However, there are still deaths in childhood, adolescence and, as in Sharon's case, early adulthood. The main causes are infections and sickling in certain parts of the body such as the spleen and lungs. Bereavement counselling is generally inadequate and the grief of mothers and other members of the family is made more acute as a result.

More recently, some patients have been cured through bone marrow transplantation, particularly in Europe (Belgium and France). This is just beginning to be considered in Britain. However, it can be a very dangerous procedure and can lead to death or severe chronic complications. A matching donor is required, preferably a brother or sister.

SICKLE CELL ANAEMIA IN WOMEN

Complications that can occur in adults include damage to the eyes, hips and shoulders. Women with sickle cell anaemia can have children and the pregnancy can go smoothly. However, it may trigger complications such as the painful crisis, anaemia or premature delivery, as well as clots in the lungs and legs. Here is Margaret's account of her two pregnancies and the impact on her and her partner:

I have two beautiful healthy children, even though I was led to believe that women with sickle cell couldn't conceive.

My pregnancies were very hard. During the first I had a massive crisis which meant that I had to have several blood transfusions. My second was easier, because I knew how to cope this time. But three months after giving birth I had a crisis which caused my kidneys to bleed for three weeks. I feel inadequate as a mother because I have sickle cell. I'm unable to give my children all that I'd like to, because I'm always in and out of hospital. But I've taught them to be self-reliant, and I'm sure this has made them stronger. When I'm not at home, Owen (my partner) looks after them, with help from our parents. He's been wonderful – so supportive. I sometimes feel I don't deserve him. He's a musician, so my sudden admissions to hospital disrupt his career. And when I'm having a crisis, he can't even cuddle me.

Margaret notes that she was led to believe, incorrectly, that women with sickle cell couldn't conceive. They therefore need information not only about pregnancy but also about contraception. It can be a two-edged sword, with some health professionals actively discouraging women from having children, while women who wish to use contraceptives are given extremely confused advice, as revealed in a recent study (Howard *et al*, 1993). The research, undertaken in 1990 and 1991, involved interviewing 149 women in London with sickle cell disorders who were aged between 18 and 48 years. At some time or other 67 (45 per cent) had used the combined oral contraceptive pill with 15 contraceptive failures and 8 discontinued because of side-effects; 30 (20 per cent) the progesterone-only pill with 6 failures and 2 discontinued due to side-effects; 26 (17 per cent) had at some time used Depo-provera with no failures and 3 discontinued because of side-effects; 28 (19 per cent) had used the IUCD (coil), with 6 failures and none discontinued. Finally 63 (42 per cent) had at some time used barrier methods such as the cap: 5 discontinued because of side-effects and there were 9 failures; 14 (9 per cent) were sterilised, one of whom reported severe regret. No thromboembolic complications such as clots in the legs or lungs

were reported. The women reported patchy and often conflicting sources of advice on family planning, both when
they wanted to start a pregnancy, and when they wanted to
avoid pregnancy. All would have welcomed more positive
advice about planning pregnancy. Sharon learned of her
pregnancy this way:

> Last April I had a very bad crisis. I was rushed to hospital
> and my haemoglobin was 3g. I was extremely yellow, very
> jaundiced. I was taken to intensive care, where they pumped
> eight units of blood into me. I was on a lot of antibiotics,
> I was very sick and I lost a lot of weight. A couple of
> months after that I became sick again; a lot of tests were
> done and no one knew what the matter with me was.
> Everything showed up negative, and then I was found to be
> pregnant – which I was shocked about but I think that
> might have sparked off my bad crisis last April. I am amazed
> that my daughter has come out so perfect, because of all
> I went through. She is a picture of health; she only has the
> trait so she is fine.
>
> *From* 'A Personal View of Sickle Cell Pain'

It is often wrongly assumed that children of affected
individuals like Margaret and Sharon will automatically
inherit sickle cell anaemia. Their children are not affected ·
because their partners do not have the trait or the illness.
They will, however, inherit sickle cell trait, which will not
turn into sickle cell anaemia. If their partners had sickle cell
trait, then there would be a 50–50 chance that all of their
children could inherit either sickle cell anaemia or sickle
cell trait. If both parents have sickle cell anaemia, then all
their children will inherit the same illness.

TESTING THE UNBORN BABY (PRENATAL DIAGNOSIS)

It is now possible to test the unborn baby for sickle cell anaemia from as early as 9–10 weeks into pregnancy. This presents a major dilemma for women and their partners when they discover that they are at risk of having a child with the condition. If the test shows that the unborn baby does have sickle cell anaemia the couple have to decide whether to terminate or continue with the pregnancy. Women are usually confronted with this agonising decision because they may be found to have sickle cell trait following a blood test in pregnancy. They are not always routinely informed about this test and so the result may come as a tremendous shock. They may have little information in the form of leaflets to help them explain to their partner why he should have a test to see if he too has the trait.

Macho attitudes can result in a furious response towards the woman for daring to suggest there could be anything 'wrong with his blood'. Even if the partner is supportive he may be frightened of having a blood test, leaving the woman in a more confused state as to whether or not they are at risk of having an affected child. If a woman knows how common sickle cell trait is in the Afro-Caribbean and West African communities her anxiety level during the pregnancy can be very high if her partner refuses to have a test or is not available. This is how one mother describes the chain of events leading up to her partner accepting *his* son's diagnosis:

> His dad said 'nobody in my family has it . . . ' But at least he went; still with a chip on his shoulder. Because Elizabeth gave me a form to give him. And then when he came back afterwards he said 'see, he's not mine! Because I ain't got nothing.' But what they'd done: at the bottom, they'd scribbled thalassaemia trait. So obviously I'm telling him he's got *sickle cell* trait – because to get sickle cell anaemia the two of us have got to have it. So then I took him down to

the Sickle Cell Society and Elizabeth patiently explained it.
So that's when we found out that he had *thalassaemia trait*
and they changed his card again. (Black and Laws, 1986)

However, even if the couple do find out that they both have
sickle cell trait, testing the unborn baby carries a risk of
miscarriage as well as the occasional mistake in diagnosis.
The fear of the test itself, as well as risking the loss of the
pregnancy as a result of the procedure, may be the deciding
factor in choosing not to have the test. Terminating a pregnancy may also be against their religious, cultural or health
beliefs. Some women are keen to have the test as they cannot
accept the risk of having a child with the illness. They may
feel that the 25 per cent risk of an affected child outweighs
the 1–2 per cent risk of miscarriage due to the test. Their decision to have the test may be influenced by their personal
knowledge of the illness, perhaps if they have already had a
seriously affected child, or as a result of experiencing the
death of someone with the illness. On the other hand, the
unpredictable and variable nature of sickle cell anaemia
makes it very difficult for women and their partners to decide
whether the condition is so severe as to warrant terminating
an affected pregnancy. There may be conflict within the
partnership, one wanting to have the test, the other adamant
that they should not. Women may also be put under considerable pressure by health professionals, families and friends
either to have the test or not. Once the decision is made, they
may not be given the support they need, whatever they have
decided.

What is scandalous is the poor level of information and
counselling available to many women who find themselves
in this situation. The recent discovery of the cystic fibrosis
gene (a condition which is mainly found amongst white
people; one in 25 white British are carriers) has generated
much interest in dilemmas that may be posed by screening
people before or during pregnancy. (An example is the

71

regular coverage in the *Observer*, for instance a full-page article by Robin McKie in the issue of 28 June 1992.) I am angered by the failure to give similar coverage to the dilemmas and needs of black women screened in the National Health Service.

Likewise, little coverage has been given in the media to positive developments taking place within the NHS. These are led in the main by black women, often nurses, who have been campaigning to develop non-directive information and counselling services. These provide women and their partners with information on conditions such as sickle cell anaemia and the tests that are available so that they can make up their own minds about whether to accept them or not. Counselling provides an opportunity to discuss the outcomes of all the options available. This approach avoids putting pressure on the woman and her partner to make a particular choice that the health professional may feel is 'responsible'. In addition, the various sickle cell support groups have been waging a difficult fight to put, and keep, sickle cell on the political agenda.

PUTTING SICKLE CELL ON THE HEALTH AGENDA

The experiences of Margaret, Sharon and others have led black health workers and support groups to campaign for better awareness and more sensitive services. The main issue is the failure of health authorities to recognise the condition as a significant health issue. The first information and counselling centre did not open until 1979, despite at least twenty years' experience of sickle cell patients in British hospitals. Even today, nearly fifteen years later, only twenty-four health authorities (there are 200 in total) have developed some kind of counselling service, some on short-term funds and with part-time staff. There is no accurate number of cases of sickle cell disorders in Britain, but an often-quoted estimate is 5,000. This is probably an underestimate as it was calculated by using as a baseline the Brent sickle cell register of the mid-1980s. Even so this number is similar to the number of cases of cystic fibrosis and haemophilia, which receive more publicity and funding. There are constant complaints from black families about poor treatment in hospital, inadequate education and information as well as failure to offer comprehensive support. Women are usually the main carers and are at the receiving end of ignorant and/or uninterested doctors, nurses, social workers, housing officers, teachers and social security officers. Complaints by families, patients, support groups and health workers led the government to ask the Standing Medical Advisory Committee to set up a working party to develop guidelines for health authorities in order to develop better services. Membership of this working party (which began meeting in 1992) includes a woman with sickle cell anaemia, myself as well as both specialist and non-specialist doctors. I see it as one chance for affected families, support groups, community workers and concerned health workers to point out present deficiencies and make recommendations for improvements.

It would be foolish to expect too much from one committee, so it is encouraging to see the increase in local support groups throughout the country and wider coverage in the black and minority ethnic media. The national sickle cell organisations have also started to meet on a regular basis, in response to a call for more unity by affected families and supporters. A confederation of sickle groups will be vital to exert sufficient political pressure for resources to be released, for better treatment, research and support for sufferers from sickle cell anaemia. The need for such support and the positive impact of greater knowledge is illustrated in this final quote from Margaret:

When I was younger, and was rushed screaming to the casualty department in crisis, I often feared that I might die. I remember several occasions when I asked my mum to bring the whole family to see me, so I could say goodbye. The nurses told me to stop screaming as I was upsetting all the other patients. I'll never forget that. They just didn't understand that pain could be so bad. But after a while people became more sympathetic as they began to be more aware of what sickle cell anaemia was.

References

Anionwu, E. N. (1988) 'Community Development and Health Education for Sickle Cell Disorders in Brent', PhD thesis, Institute of Education, University of London.

Anionwu, E. N. (in press) 'Sickle Cell and Thalassaemia – Community Struggles and Official Response', in W. Ahmad (ed.), *'Race' & Health in Contemporary Britain*, Milton Keynes, Open University Press.

Black, J. and Laws, S. (1986) *Living with Sickle Cell Disease*, London, Sickle Cell Society.

Deacon, M. (1991) 'Coping with Sickle Cell Anaemia', *Woman's Own*, 25 March, 25–6.

Edwards, S. 'A Personal View of Sickle Cell Pain', in Shanklemen, J. and May, A., *Pain in Sickle Cell Disease, Setting Standards of Care*, March 1993, Cardiff Sickle Cell and Thalassemia Centre.

Howard, R. J., Lillis, C. and Tuck, S. M. (1993) 'Contraceptives Counselling and Pregnancy in Women With Sickle Cell Disease', *British Medical Journal*, Vol. 306, pp 1735–7.

Further Suggested Reading

Anionwu, E. N. and Jibril, H. (1986) *Sickle Cell Disease – A Guide for Families*, London, Collins.

Franklin, I (1990) *Sickle Cell Disease. A Guide for Patients, Carers and Health Workers*, London, Faber & Faber.

Serjeant, G. R. (1992) *Sickle Cell Disease*, Oxford, Oxford University Press, 2nd edition.

Sickle Cell Society (1992) *Sickle Cell Disease – The Need for Improved Services*, London, Sickle Cell Society, 3rd edition.

Black Women and HIV/AIDS

Nozipho Patricia January-Bardill

Much of the recent evidence about AIDS points to the increasing spread of HIV amongst women. The World Health Organisation (WHO) has predicted that by the end of the century there will be an estimated 40 million cases of HIV globally. Ninety per cent of these cases will be spread through heterosexual contact; and women who are HIV positive will outnumber HIV-positive men. In Britain, the number of new HIV cases in women rose by 27 per cent in the year up to September 1991, compared to 8 per cent for men (Sadgrove, 1992). Black and Latino women and children constitute about 80 per cent of all cases of AIDS in the United States.

But statistics alone do not necessarily provide explanations for specific trends in the spread of HIV, nor do they offer solutions. The historical association of HIV with white, gay men, combined with social, economic and political factors that include, for example, class, race and gender, must play a major part in any analysis of the impact of HIV on different social groups.

WOMEN AND AIDS
Though the situation is changing slowly (most often as

75

a result of work done by women), it is still the case primarily that women are not an essential part of the discussions that surround the transmission, diagnosis, research, treatment and care of those living with HIV and AIDS. Margaret Jay, ex-director of the National AIDS Trust, has noted that 'only recently have the particular concerns of women infected and affected by the HIV virus been acknowledged and openly discussed'.[1]

> There has been very little analysis of the experience of women who are antibody positive or who have AIDS and there is still only a small voice heard from those women who are most profoundly affected by the virus. As with so many other societal issues, we are in danger of extrapolating from the male situation to the female, and this is neither tenable nor indeed possible. Women's access to health care, the support systems available to them, their ability to make changes in their sex lives and their reactions to physical decline and disfigurement, are likely to be different from men's.[2]

The mechanics of the sexual transmission of HIV are such that men appear to pass on HIV more effectively than women during unprotected or vaginal and anal intercourse. Research indicates that women are twice as likely to be infected by men than men by women. Despite these observations women are increasingly becoming the targets of blame for spreading HIV. For example, it is female prostitutes, and not their male punters, who have been accused of spreading HIV. They have been easy fodder for many scientific and medical researchers who have unashamedly invaded their lives. Numerous reports and accounts have been written about prostitutes and HIV. Save for self-help initiatives by prostitutes themselves, however, very little has been done to improve the quality of their lives.

The position of poor women in both 'developed' and 'developing' countries has also been ignored. The sexism of those who control the medical establishment is manifested in several ways:

- It is generally accepted that there is a lack of clear gynaecological information in the official definition of HIV and AIDS (though vaginal thrush, for example, is very common in women with HIV infection) (Bury, *et al.*1992).
- Not enough information exists about woman-to-woman transmission.
- Women are either mis-diagnosed or under-diagnosed and die of HIV-related illnesses much faster than men. According to one study, a woman with AIDS can expect to live only for between 15 weeks and six months after diagnosis, compared with 24 to 36 weeks for a man. ACT-UP, the international AIDS activist group, reports that many women in the US die of AIDS-Related Complex (ARC) and concludes that the guidelines for an AIDS diagnosis clearly overlook the patterns of HIV disease in women (ACT-UP, 1990).
- Under-diagnosis and mis-diagnosis mean that women have less access to treatment and welfare benefits which are specifically for people with HIV and AIDS.
- Many experimental drug trials have in the past excluded all women, including black women, who are current and ex-drug users, poor women, young women and girls.

As AIDS has taken hold as a worldwide epidemic, it has become increasingly clear that women *are* affected by HIV and AIDS – and not just as wives, mothers, sisters, aunts, etc. of men with HIV and AIDS – and that descriptions of the disease in terms solely of its effects on gay men are inaccurate and misleading. However, social implications of HIV for women cannot be examined in isolation from the position of women in society. For so many women who are infected and affected, their position is characterised by financial and emotional dependence, which is reinforced by the legal system, the health care system and social services.[3]

BLACK WOMEN AND HIV/AIDS

Information aimed at black women with HIV/AIDS is noticeable by its absence. This is a very curious situation when you consider that in New York City, for example, 'the bulk of the women being infected are poor minority women', who are drug users sharing unsterilised injection equipment.[4] In Britain, evidence suggests that black women are more likely to be tested without their knowledge or consent. Despite this, it is difficult to find information specifically directed towards black women with HIV/AIDS.

This lack of information about HIV prevention and care raises questions about access to services and treatment. The consequences for black women have been delayed diagnosis and treatment of HIV infection and AIDS, a situation regularly observed by the Black HIV and AIDS Network (BHAN). BHAN is a national organisation set up in 1988–9 to respond to the needs of African, Caribbean and Asian communities affected by HIV and AIDS. According to BHAN's observations, as well as those of many social services departments and hospitals, black women and children present late with severe HIV disease because fear and stigma about the condition prevent them from accepting and approaching HIV services.

A report by Hammersmith and Fulham social services department, for example, notes that

women are presenting in increasing numbers, but very often in much later stages of the illness. This appears to be particularly so for black women from some African countries, who are here as refugees or who have settled in the United Kingdom over the past few years. Some women suffer the double disadvantage of both the illness and media/public prejudice that seeks to 'blame' African people for the spread of the disease and they may therefore be reluctant to approach services that do not demonstrate sensitivity to their particular needs.[5]

Trends observed in the US also indicate that black women seem to develop AIDS faster than white women and men. The average survival time for a black woman in New York is around fifteen days after an AIDS diagnosis, and less than eight weeks for a white woman in San Francisco (Sadgrove, 1992):

> A number of studies of survival of people with AIDS have found that women survive a significantly shorter time after a diagnosis of AIDS than men and Black women drug users survive the shortest time of all . . . Shorter survival in women could be due to a number of factors. AIDS sometimes takes a much slower course in men who present with Kaposi's sarcoma which is a rare presentation in women. Women tend to come forward later in the disease than men, particularly in the US where they have poorer access to health care due to poverty. Poor and minority women in particular are unlikely to be receiving ongoing preventative medical care and may be reluctant to seek help when they are ill.[6]

Besides a lack of information and the fear of being stigmatised or ostracised, other factors affecting black women with HIV/AIDS include racism in the NHS; inappropriate medical advice and mis-diagnosis; serious social and economic difficulties; and family and domestic commitments. BHAN has experienced numerous cases of black women who are totally at a loss as to how to manage their lives after a diagnosis of HIV:

> Sarah knew she was ill, but her doctor dismissed her because she did not 'look ill'. He prescribed doses of antibiotics without diagnosing her symptoms.
>
> Linda did not know she had HIV-related symptoms. She found out about her status after her child had been tested without her consent.
>
> *BHAN case files*

The physical, social and psychological burdens for black women living with HIV and AIDS and who have young children and other dependants are also heightened. Black women are often the main source of care, so greater demands are made on their energies and resources:

> Elizabeth was ill with AIDS and had come to terms with the fact that she did not have long to live. Her main concern was to ensure that her three children were well cared for. Her plans to secure a future for the children were frustrated by the fact that no one could meet her specific needs. Existing services expected her to fit into pre-planned formulae which conflicted with her needs. Despite her very task oriented approach to dealing with her predicament, she felt frustrated and angry.
>
> *BHAN case files*

Social services and the white AIDS voluntary sector do not always meet the needs of black women. For example, one of the initiatives which emerged from gay men's struggles against AIDS was the notion of support groups. While these worked well for a certain class of white, gay men, support groups proved less popular with black women. They preferred to maintain their anonymity, not because they didn't want to associate with others, but because of the stigma associated with HIV, particularly community attitudes to it, and, in the case of refugee women, the implications for obtaining asylum status.

Hospital appointments are another case in point. Black

women are often forced to miss appointments for any number of personal reasons, for example family commitments, problems of transport, or ill-health. Seldom are attempts made to find out why they have been unable to attend. Anecdotal evidence suggests, however, that assumptions are made about them, which results in their being labelled as negligent or careless. Needs assessment is therefore made on the basis of erroneous or sometimes no information. BHAN has found that district and community nurses in some health authorities are not mobilised to support the women adequately. Often women go to hospital for short stays, yet little is done to co-ordinate services which the women can then utilise when they return home. Crisis management becomes the norm for managing the woman's illness.

These problems are even more acute for black women whose first language is not English. They have particular difficulty in trying to understand the facts about HIV and AIDS, as well as the distinct roles of their assigned carers. One local authority social services department in London regularly assigns social work students to black women living with HIV disease. The fact that it takes time to assess a person, build a relationship and organise care seems to be overlooked. Many people living with AIDS are weary of repeating their life experiences to several different people and would appreciate a sense of continuity in their care.

Money is also a major problem for black women living with HIV and AIDS. Black women who are students often have to drop out of their education, with no access to welfare benefits or housing. Existing from day to day can be quite traumatic. Malnutrition is not uncommon for black women and this of course leads to more rapid onset of illness.

Although information on welfare benefits is readily available, the workers at BHAN have found that forms can be unnecessarily complicated. Women from refugee communities often lose out on benefits: they are either reluctant to claim or often do not understand how the system works. In addition, some in the medical establishment still use the African connection to infringe on the human and civil rights of black women.

> Terry was pregnant. She went to hospital for the usual ante-natal care and was given a form – one routinely given to pregnant women at a number of hospitals in London. The form categorically states that 'high risk' groups for selective HIV testing (as defined by the Department of Health AIDS Unit) includes 'Women who have had sex at any time since 1977 with people living in African countries, except those on the Mediterranean, or who have sexual partners who have done so.'
>
> *BHAN case files*

The obvious question is why those who have had sex with people living in America at any time since 1977 are excluded from the 'high-risk' category, if indeed such categories are justifiable. Terry is not continental African, but black British. She felt stigmatised and annoyed. The sub-text is that black people are more promiscuous and are actively spreading HIV.

In a number of cases black women have been refused minor surgery unless they agree to have an HIV test:

> Susan phoned to speak to someone about a consultant who refused to give her a D&C (dilation and curettage) because he insisted that she had an HIV test first. She was aware of her rights and refused to have the test. She was told to go to another hospital which was miles away from where she lived.
>
> *BHAN case files*

The plight of black women living with HIV highlights the kind of institutional racism which is typical of some parts of the health and social services. The history of racism with regard to mental health in black communities, along with inadequate responses to the treatment of sickle cell anaemia and thalassaemia, are further examples. These latter two conditions are hardly mentioned in HIV and AIDS discourse, despite their association with blood transfusions.

NATIONAL AND LOCAL RESPONSES

Although the Department of Health's circular, *HIV and AIDS: Resource Allocation 1989/90*, requires health authorities to set up services which are targeted at groups with specific needs, there is still little evidence that much is being done at national, district and local levels to respond to the needs of black communities and black women. In addition the leaflets, posters and other prevention materials which do exist are generally of a poor quality.

The National Health Service in Britain offers black people relatively better access to health care than is available in America. However, many white health carers and social workers are afraid or reluctant to take responsibility for organising the care of black clients with HIV. Direct and indirect racism, fears about not getting it right and an inability to relate to black people generally accounts for much of the tentative behaviour towards black clients.

Although the Department of Health is encouraging agencies to adopt collaborative approaches to health and social care, different agencies often have conflicting philosophies and approaches to treatment and care. Local authorities, for example, have been battling to implement equal opportunities policies targeted at groups who have faced discrimination for several years, and though there are not enough visible outcomes to measure their success, they are relatively better equipped to address issues of race or class than health sector workers, many of whom still believe that the colour-blind approach of treating everyone the same is the only way to respond to the health needs of individuals.

Black HIV/AIDS organisations in the voluntary sector such as BHAN, Blackliners, the Black HIV/AIDS Forums (BHAF) in Leicester, Leeds, Birmingham and Manchester are examples of voluntary organisations that are working with very limited resources to address the issues which HIV has raised for black people. BHAN has excelled in the organisation of care for black people, and particularly black women living with HIV and AIDS. It has offered counselling in languages other than English and has developed a holistic model of care that attempts to meet the medical, social, material and spiritual needs of clients.

THE NEED FOR A NEW PERSPECTIVE ON BLACK WOMEN'S HEALTH

It is clear that HIV has highlighted distinctions of race, class, gender and sexuality in a way that no other health-related condition has done in the past. There is therefore a need to re-examine the way in which the general health of oppressed groups coincides with their power in any society.

Health and disease are products of the way in which, amongst others, sexuality, reproduction, childrearing, work and socialisation are organised. An analysis of the state of health of any society must include health education, nutrition, mental health, the organisation of health care as well as the impact of social, economic, political, ideological and legal systems (Turshen, 1989).

The distribution of resources that are vital for black women's health such as access to adequate housing, food, social and welfare services, is a function of the relative power of the white people who control these terrains and black people who don't. Those who are in control of the health and medical services are socialised and educated to think in terms of the biological and environmental causes of disease rather than the social production of illness. Black people are often accused of having a chip on their shoulder or labelled as schizophrenic if they associate their ill-health or depression with racism, poverty and unemployment.

Those who control the social services sometimes confuse social care with social control. They also treat people from different classes and races unequally. It has been interesting to observe how easily white middle-class men living with HIV who do not have a history with social care organisations have accessed social services. Black and white working-class people with HIV, who have had a more chequered history with social services departments and have been at the receiving end of the controlling elements of social services, have not always had the same ease of access and care. A number of black people with HIV are referred to the black voluntary organisations by social workers. BHAN has several case histories to illustrate this point.

Black women do not control the institutions that affect their health and well-being. On the contrary, the objective social reality of black women is that they are at the bottom of the social pecking order in the UK. The fact that so little is known about the specific ways in which HIV affects women; the fact that so few black women manage health services generally and HIV services specifically in this country; the fact that black women are seldom asked to participate in decisions that affect their well-being but are instead pathologised and labelled irresponsible, strong and hard, all contribute to the despair and powerlessness that they sometimes feel.

Until these issues are addressed seriously the tendency to observe and respond to symptoms rather than causes of disease and illness will continue. HIV and AIDS are a public health issue. A holistic approach which takes into account the socio-economic circumstances of people's lives must enter the discussion concerning the care of those infected with the virus as well as prevention strategies to stop the spread of HIV.

FUTURE STRATEGIES FOR BLACK WOMEN

While the NHS is a better health system than the more commercial approach to health in the US (it is cheaper and accessible to more people), recent reforms to purchase and contract health care from so-called providers are bound to have a serious impact on the more disenfranchised members of this society, of which black people and particularly women, are a part. Contract specifications often exclude criteria that relate to equity of services.

A holistic approach by both the health and social welfare sectors which includes, for example, material, social, recreational and emotional factors in assessing the health needs of black women will go a long way to discovering the real causes of some of the questions related to the short life expectancy of women with HIV. By using this approach BHAN soon learned that whole families were affected by HIV. Poverty, homelessness, transcontinental support systems, unemployment and many other social and economic considerations had to be addressed to provide the most appropriate service for people living with HIV and AIDS. BHAN had to respond very quickly by adapting to a family-centred as well as an individualised approach to service provision.

Black women will need to continue to lobby against discrimination and demand:

- more participation in policy development in health, social and welfare services; and the production of information on HIV and AIDS.
- better ethical practices which genuinely respect the rights of black women and acknowledge the need to treat them with dignity;
- a more efficient and confidential counselling service;
- more respite care facilities, as well as organised family and home care services;
- more time to plan their own care and that of dependants;

- flexible services instead of predetermined formulas for dealing with problems;
- more support from district nurses and health visitors with clearer explanations of different professionals' roles, to maximise patient care;
- a bigger role in identifying women's own needs and maintaining control over their lives. HIV has, besides other things, highlighted the limitations of clinical medicine both in the way people's lives get taken over by doctors and also in the way treatments are administered to patients.
- good interpreters and translators who understand HIV and all related issues for women whose first language is not English;
- HIV prevention education which is user friendly to black women. The use of radio, outreach and other community development approaches needs to be explored and tested. Black women are not a homogeneous group, and prevention strategies need to bear this in mind;
- more appropriate information and better sex education targeted at young black women;
- safer sex information that does not overlook the power dimensions of sexual decision-making as well as the social, religious and cultural values which underpin black women's lives;
- space to develop our own understanding of HIV and AIDS and address it within the context of our social, economic, cultural and political experience;
- an awareness that black women are women first rather than mothers, partners and carers only;
- more networking by black voluntary and self-help women's organisations;
- better collaborative work between statutory and voluntary agencies which are serious about promoting the health needs of black people, and black women specifically.

The positive side-effect of HIV is that it has forced us all to address hitherto hidden issues like sex and sexuality, drug use, prostitution, and death and dying. It presents us with a chance to reclaim our sexuality, take control of our bodies, stop making decisions which put our lives at risk, and take a more active role in personal relations between ourselves and men. The caring role of black women has led to the denial of our own dependency needs. We often find it hard to ask for help. While Maya Angelou rightly observes our ability to rise in the face of adversity, our health needs will demand that we rest and sometimes take time out for ourselves.

Notes

Thanks to Sophie Johnson of the Black HIV and AIDS Network for her patience, time and total commitment to providing the best possible care for black people living with HIV and AIDS in London.

1. M. Jay, in *Working with Women and AIDS*, London, Routledge, 1992, p. xiii.
2. J. Barlow, 'Social Issues, an Overview', ibid., p. 23.
3. Ibid.
4. E. Springer, 'Reflections on Women and HIV/AIDS in New York City and the United States', ibid., p. 34.
5. *Social Services Committee Report*, Hammersmith and Fulham Council, January 1993.
6. J. Bury, 'Women and the AIDS Epidemic: Some Medical Facts and Figures', in *Working with Women and AIDS*, op. cit., p. 19.

References

ACT Up/New York (1990) *Women, AIDS and Activism*, Boston, Mass., South End Press.
AIDS Newsletter (1992) 7 (8) June, London, Bureau of Hygiene and Tropical Diseases.
Bhatt, C. (1991) *AIDS and the Black Communities* (BHAN Policy Report 1), London, Camden Council.
Bhatt, C. (1992) 'Empowerment and Understanding. HIV Prevention Work with Black Minority Ethnic Communities', in *Working Where the Risks Are*, London, Health Education Authority.

Bury, J., Morrison, V., and McLachlan, S. (1992) 'Women and the AIDS Epidemic: Some Medical Facts and Figures', *Working with Women and AIDS*, London, Routledge.

Department of Health (1992) *Allocation for HIV and AIDS Work*, Department of Health, London.

January-Bardill, N. P. (1991) 'HIV/AIDS in Africa: A Public Health Perspective', *Africa World Review*, London, African Research & Information Bureau.

Sadgrove, J. (1992) *Women with AIDS*, London, Vogue, 1992.

Turshen, M. (1989) *The Politics of Public Health*, London, Zed Books.

Living With Cancer

....

Audre Lorde

For the past several decades, black women have consistently had a 12–15 per cent poorer five-year survival rate from breast cancer than white women. While black women develop breast cancer less frequently than white women, more of us die from the disease – primarily because we do not receive adequate health care. Studies show that you can help reduce your cancer risk by stopping smoking, improving your diet and conducting regular breast self-examinations.

7 June 1984
Berlin
Dr Rosenberg agrees with my decision not to have a biopsy, but she has said I must do something quickly to strengthen my bodily defences. She's recommended I begin Iscador injections three times weekly.

Iscador is a biological made from mistletoe which strengthens the natural immune system, and works against the growth of malignant cells. I've started the injections, along with two other herbals that stimulate liver function. I feel less weak.

I am listening to what fear teaches. I will never be gone. I am a scar, a report from the frontlines, a talisman, a resurrection. A rough place on the chin of complacency . . .

So what if I am afraid? Of stepping out into the morning? Of dying? Of unleashing the dammed gall where hatred swims like a tadpole waiting to swell into the arms of war? And what does that war teach when the bruised leavings jump an insurmountable wall where the glorious Berlin chestnuts and orange poppies hide detection wires that spray bullets which kill?

My poems are filled with blood these days because the future is so bloody. When the blood of four-year-old children runs unremarked through the alleys of Soweto, how can I pretend that sweetness is anything more than armour and ammunition in an ongoing war?

I am saving my life by using my life in the service of what must be done. Tonight as I listened to the African National Congress speakers from South Africa at the Third World People's Center here, I was filled with a sense of self-answering necessity, of commitment as a survival weapon. Our battles are inseparable. Every person I have ever been must be actively enlisted in those battles, as well as in the battle to save my life.

9 June 1984
Berlin
At the poetry reading in Zurich this weekend, I found it so much easier to discuss racism than to talk about *The Cancer Journals*. Chemical plants between Zurich and Basle have been implicated in a definite rise in breast cancer in this region, and women wanted to discuss this. I talked as honestly as I could, but it was really hard. Their questions presume a clarity I no longer have.

It was great to have Gloria there to help field all those questions about racism. For the first time in Europe, I felt I was not alone but answering as one of a group of Black women – not just Audre Lorde!

I am cultivating every iota of my energies to do battle with the possibility of liver cancer. At the same time, I am discovering how furious and resistant some pieces of me are, as well as how terrified.

In this loneliest of places, I examine every decision I make within the light of what I've learned about myself and that self-destructiveness implanted inside of me by racism and sexism and the circumstances of my life as a Black woman.

> Mother why were we armed to fight
> with cloud wreathed swords and javelins of dust?

Survival isn't some theory operating in a vacuum. It's a matter of my everyday living and making decisions.

How do I hold faith with the sun in a sunless place? It is so hard not to counter this despair with a refusal to see. But I have to stay open and filtering no matter what's coming at me, because that arms me in a particularly Black woman's way. When I'm open I'm also less despairing. The more clearly I see what I'm up against, the more able I am to fight this process going on in my body that they're calling liver cancer. And I am determined to fight it even when I am not sure of the terms of the battle nor the face of victory. I just know I must not surrender my body to others unless I completely understand and agree with what they think should be done to it. I've got to look at all of my options carefully, even the ones I find distasteful. I know I can broaden the definition of winning to the point where I can't lose.

10 June 1984
Berlin
Dr Rosenberg is honest, straightforward, and pretty discouraging. I don't know what I'd do without Dagmar there to translate all her grim pronouncements for me. She thinks it's liver cancer, too, but she respects my decision against surgery. I mustn't let my unwillingness to accept this diagnosis interfere with getting help. Whatever it is, this seems to be working.

We all have to die at least once. Making that death useful would be winning for me. I wasn't supposed to exist anyway, not in any meaningful way in this fucked-up whiteboys' world. I want desperately to live, and I'm ready to fight for that living even if I die shortly. Just writing those words down snaps everything I want to do into a neon clarity. This European trip and the Afro-German women, the Sister Outsider collective in Holland, Gloria's great idea of starting an organisation that can be a connection between us and South African women. For the first time I really feel that my writing has a substance and stature that will survive me.

I have done good work. I see it in the letters that come to me about *Sister Outsider*. I see it in the use women here give the poetry and the prose. But first and last I am a poet. I've worked very hard for that approach to living inside myself, and everything I do, I hope, reflects that view of life, even the ways I must move now in order to save my life.

I have done good work. There is a hell of a lot more I have to do. And sitting here tonight in this lovely green park in Berlin, dusk approaching and the walking willows leaning over the edge of the pool caressing each other's fingers, birds birds birds singing under and over the frogs, and the smell of new-mown grass enveloping my sad pen, I feel I still have enough moxie to do it all, on whatever terms I'm dealt, timely or not. Enough moxie to chew the whole world up and spit it out in bite-sized pieces, useful and warm and wet and delectable because they came out of my mouth.

17 June 1984
Berlin
I am feeling more like an Audre I recognise, thank the goddess for Dr Rosenberg, and for Dagmar for introducing me to her.

I've been reading Christa Wolf's *The Search for Christa T.* and finding it very difficult. At first I couldn't grapple with it because it was too painful to read about a woman dying. Dagmar and a number of the women here in Berlin say the author and I should meet. But now that I'm finished I don't know if I want to meet the woman who wrote it. There is so much pain there that is so far from being felt in any way I recognise or can use, that it makes me very uncomfortable. I feel speechless.

But there is one part of the book that really spoke to me. In chapter five she talks about a mistaken urge to laugh at one's younger self's belief in paradise, in miracles. Each one of us who survives, she says, at least once in our lifetime, at some crucial and inescapable moment, has had to absolutely believe in the impossible. Of course, it occurs to me to ask myself if that's what I'm doing right now, believing in the impossible by refusing a biopsy.

It's been very reassuring to find a medical doctor who agrees with my view of the dangers involved. And I certainly don't reject non-damaging treatment, which is why I'm taking these shots, even though I hate giving myself injections. But that's a small price balanced against the possibility of cancer.

8 November 1986
New York City
If I am to put this all down in a way that is useful, I should start with the beginning of the story.

Sizeable tumour in the right lobe of the liver, the doctors said. Lots of blood vessels in it means it's most likely malignant. Let's cut you open right now and see what we can do about it. Wait a minute, I said. I need to feel this thing out and see what's going on inside myself first, I said, needing some time to absorb the shock, time to assay the situation and not act out of panic. Not one of them said, I can respect that, but don't take too long about it.

94

Instead, that simple claim to my body's own processes elicited such an attack response from a reputable Specialist in Liver Tumours that my deepest — if not necessarily most useful — suspicions were totally aroused.

What that doctor could have said to me that I would have heard was, 'You have a serious condition going on in your body and whatever you do about it you must not ignore it or delay deciding how you are going to deal with it because it will not go away no matter what you think it is.' Acknowledging my responsibility for my own body. Instead, what he said to me was, 'If you do not do exactly what I tell you to do right now without questions you are going to die a horrible death.' In exactly those words.

I felt the battle lines being drawn up within my own body.

I saw this specialist in liver tumours at a leading cancer hospital in New York City, where I had been referred as an outpatient by my own doctor.

The first people who interviewed me in white coats from behind a computer were only interested in my health care benefits and proposed method of payment. Those crucial facts determined what kind of plastic identification card I would be given, and without a plastic ID card, no one at all was allowed upstairs to see any doctor, as I was told by the uniformed, pistolled guards at all the stairwells.

From the moment I was ushered into the doctor's office and he saw my X-rays, he proceeded to infantilise me with an obviously well-practised technique. When I told him I was having second thoughts about a liver biopsy, he glanced at my chart. Racism and Sexism joined hands across his table as he saw I taught at a university. 'Well, you look like an *intelligent girl*,' he said, staring at my one breast all the time he was speaking. 'Not to have this biopsy immediately is like sticking your head in the sand.' Then he went on to say that he would not be responsible when I wound up one day screaming in agony in the corner of his office!

I asked this specialist in liver tumours about the dangers of a liver biopsy spreading an existing malignancy, or even encouraging it in a borderline tumour. He dismissed my concerns with a wave of his hand, saying, instead of answering, that I really did not have any other sensible choice.

I would like to think that this doctor was sincerely motivated by a desire for me to seek what he truly believed to be the only remedy for my sickening body, but my faith in that scenario is considerably diminished by his 250-dollar consultation fee and his subsequent medical report to my own doctor containing numerous supposedly clinical observations of *obese abdomen* and *remaining pendulous breast*.

In any event, I can thank him for the fierce shard lancing through my terror that shrieked there must be some other way, this doesn't feel right to me. If this is cancer and they cut me open to find out, what is stopping that intrusive action from spreading the cancer, or turning a questionable mass into an active malignancy? All I was asking for was the reassurance of a realistic answer to my real questions, and that was not forthcoming. I made up my mind that if I was going to die in agony on somebody's office floor, it certainly wasn't going to be his! I needed information, and pored over books on the liver in Barnes & Noble's Medical Textbook Section on Fifth Avenue for hours. I learned, among other things, that the liver is the largest, most complex, and most generous organ in the human body. But that did not help me very much.

In this period of physical weakness and psychic turmoil, I found myself going through an intricate inventory of rage. First of all at my breast surgeon, had he perhaps done something wrong? How could such a small breast tumour have metastasised? Hadn't he assured me he'd gotten it all, and what was this now anyway about micro-metastases? Could this tumour in my liver have been seeded at the same time as my breast cancer? There were so many unanswered questions, and too much that I just did not understand.

But my worst rage was the rage at myself. For a brief time I felt like a total failure. What had I been busting my ass doing these past six years if it wasn't living and loving and working to my utmost potential? And wasn't that all a guarantee supposed to keep exactly this kind of thing from ever happening again? So what had I done wrong and what was I going to have to pay for it and WHY ME?

But finally a little voice inside me said sharply, 'Now really, is there any other way you would have preferred living the past six years that would have been more satisfying? And be that as it may, *should* or *shouldn't* isn't even the question. How do you want to live the rest of your life from now on and what are you going to do about it?' Time's awasting!

Gradually, in those hours in the stacks of Barnes & Noble, I felt myself shifting into another gear. My resolve strengthened as my panic lessened. Deep breathing, regularly. I'm not going to let them cut into my body again until I'm convinced there is no other alternative. And this time, the burden of proof rests with the doctors because their record of success with liver cancer is not so good that it would make me jump at a surgical solution. And scare tactics are not going to work. I have been scared now for six years and that hasn't stopped me. I've given myself plenty of practice in doing whatever I need to do, scared or not, so scare tactics are just not going to work. Or I hoped they were not going to work. At any rate, thank the goddess, they were not working yet. One step at a time.

But some of my nightmares were pure hell and I started having trouble sleeping.

In writing this I have discovered how important some things are that I thought were unimportant. I discovered this by the high price they exact for scrutiny. At first I did not want to look again at how I slowly came to terms with my own mortality on a level deeper than before, nor with the inevitable strength that it gave me as I started to get on with my life in actual time. Medical textbooks on the liver were fine, but there were appointments to be kept, and bills to pay, and decisions about my upcoming trip to Europe to be made. And what do I say to my children? Honesty has always been the bottom line between us, but did I really need them going through this with me during their final difficult years at college? On the other hand, how could I shut them out of this most important decision of my life?

I made a visit to my breast surgeon, a doctor with whom I have always been able to talk frankly, and it was from him that I got my first trustworthy and objective sense of timing. It was from him that I learned the conventional forms of treatment for liver metastases made little more than one year's difference in the survival rate. I heard my old friend Clem's voice coming back to me through the dimness of thirty years: 'I see you coming here trying to make sense where there is no sense. Try just living in it. Respond, alter, see what happens.' I thought of the African way of perceiving life, as experience to be lived rather than as a problem to be solved.

Homoeopathic medicine calls cancer the cold disease. I understand that down to my bones that quake sometimes in their need for heat, for the sun, even for just a hot bath. Part of the way in which I am saving my own life is to refuse to submit my body to cold whenever possible.

In general, I fight hard to keep my treatment scene together in some coherent and serviceable way, integrated into my daily living and absolute. Forgetting is no excuse. It's as simple as one missed shot could make the difference between a quiescent malignancy and one that is growing again. This not only keeps me in an intimate, positive relationship to my own health, but it also underlines the fact that I have the responsibility for attending my own health. I cannot simply hand over that responsibility to anybody else.

Which does not mean I give in to the belief, arrogant or naive, that I know everything I need to know in order to make informed decisions about my body. But attending my own health, gaining enough information to help me understand and participate in the decisions made about my body by people who know more medicine than I do, are all crucial strategies in my battle for living. They also provide me with important prototypes for doing battle in all other arenas of my life.

Battling racism and battling heterosexism and battling apartheid share the same urgency inside me as battling cancer. None of these struggles is ever easy, and even the smallest victory is never to be taken for granted. Each victory must be applauded, because it is so easy not to battle at all, to just accept and call that acceptance inevitable.

And all power is relative. Recognising the existence as well as the limitations of my own power, and accepting the responsibility for using it in my own behalf, involve me in direct and daily actions that preclude denial as a possible refuge. Simone de Beauvoir's words echo in my head: 'It is in the recognition of the genuine conditions of our lives that we gain the strength to act and our motivation for change.'

10 November 1986
New York City
Building into my living – without succumbing to it – an awareness of this reality of my life, that I have a condition within my body of which I will eventually die, comes in waves, like a rising tide. It exists side by side with another force inside me that says no you don't, not you, and the X-rays are wrong and the tests are wrong and the doctors are wrong.

There is a different kind of energy inherent within each one of these feelings, and I try to reconcile and use these different energies whenever I need them. The energy generated by the first awareness serves to urge me always to get on with living my life and doing my work with an intensity and purpose of the urgent now. Throw the toys overboard, we're headed for the rougher waters.

The energies generated by the second force fuel a feisty determination to continue doing what I am doing for ever. The tensions created inside me by the contradictions are another source of energy and learning. I have always known I learn my most lasting lessons about difference by closely attending the ways in which the differences in me lie together.

11 November 1986
New York City
I keep observing how other people die, comparing, learning, critiquing the process inside of me, matching it up to how I would like to do it. And I think about this scrutiny of myself in the context of its usefulness to other Black women living with cancer, born and unborn.

I have a privileged life or else I would be dead by now. It is two and a half years since the first tumour in my liver was discovered. When I needed to know, there was no one around to tell me that there were alternatives to turning myself over to doctors who are terrified of not knowing everything. There was no one around to remind me that I have a right to decide what happens to my own body, not because I know more than anybody else, but simply because it is my body. And I have a right to acquire the information that can help me make those crucial decisions.

It was an accident of circumstance that brought me to Germany at a critical moment in my health, and another which introduced me to one holistic/homoeopathic approach to the treatment of certain cancers. Not all homoeopathic alternatives work for every patient. Time is a crucial element in the treatment of cancer, and I had to decide which chances I would take, and why.

I think of what this means to other Black women living with cancer, to all women in general. Most of all I think of how important it is for us to share with each other the powers buried within the breaking of silence about our bodies and our health, even though we have been schooled to be secret and stoical about pain and disease. But that stoicism and silence do not serve us nor our communities, only the forces of things as they are.

12 November 1986
New York City
When I write my own Book of the Dead, my own Book of Life, I want to celebrate being alive to do it even while I acknowledge the painful savour uncertainty lends to my living. I use the energy of dreams that are now impossible, not totally believing in them nor their power to become real, but recognising them as templates for a future within which my labours can play a part. I am freer to choose what I will devote my energies toward and what I will leave for another lifetime, thanking the goddess for the strength to perceive that I can choose, despite obstacles.

So when I do a reading to raise funds for the women's health collectives in Soweto, or to raise money for Kitchen Table: Women of Color Press, I am choosing to use myself for things in which I passionately believe. When I speak to rally support in the urgent war against apartheid in South Africa and the racial slaughter that is even now spreading across the US, when I demand justice in the police shot-gun killing of a Black grandmother and lynchings in Northern California and in Central Park in New York City, I am making a choice of how I wish to use my power. This work gives me a tremendous amount of energy back in satisfaction and in belief, as well as in a vision of how I want this earth to be for the people who come after me.

When I work with young poets who are reaching for the power of their poetry within themselves and the lives they choose to live, I feel I am working to capacity, and this gives me deep joy, a reservoir of strength I draw upon for the next venture. Right now. This makes it far less important that it will not be for ever. It never was.

The energies I gain from my work help me neutralise those implanted forces of negativity and self-destructiveness that are white America's way of making sure I keep whatever is powerful and creative within me unavailable, ineffective, and non-threatening.

But there is a terrible clarity that comes from living with cancer that can be empowering if we do not turn aside from it. What more can they do to me? My time is limited, and this is so for each one of us. So how will the opposition reward me for my silences? For the pretence that this is in fact the best of all possible worlds? What will they give me for lying? A lifelong Safe-Conduct Pass for everyone I love? Another lifetime for me? The end to racism? Sexism? Homophobia? Cruelty? The common cold?

13 November 1986
New York City
I do not find it useful any longer to speculate upon cancer as a political weapon. But I'm not being paranoid when I say my cancer is as political as if some CIA agent brushed past me in the A train on March 15, 1965 and air-injected me with a long-fused cancer virus. Or even if it is only that I stood in their wind to do my work and the billows flayed me. What possible choices do most of us have in the air we breathe and the water we must drink?

Sometimes we are blessed with being able to choose the time and the arena and the manner of our revolution, but more usually we must do battle wherever we are standing. It does not matter too much if it is in the radiation lab or a doctor's office or the telephone company, the streets, the welfare department or the classroom. The real blessing is to be able to use whoever I am wherever I am, in concert with as many others as possible, or alone if needs be.

This is no longer a time of waiting. It is a time for the real work's urgencies. It is a time enhanced by iron reclamation of what I call the burst of light — that inescapable knowledge, in the bone, of my own physical limitations. Metabolised and integrated into the fabric of my days, that knowledge makes the particulars of what is coming seem less important. When I speak of wanting as much good time as possible, I mean time over which I maintain some relative measure of control.

Editor's Note

Sadly, Audre Lorde lost her fight against cancer in November 1992. She is greatly missed; but the survival tactics that she left for us as black women ensure that she continues to live in each of us.

One Woman's Experience of Lupus

Paula Thomas Fenton

Lupus is an illness which disproportionately affects black women. The symptoms vary from person to person. The following personal account by a black woman sufferer helps to provide an understanding of the social and psychological consequences of this disease, and sheds light on a disease which still baffles many in the medical profession.

Back in the early 1970s, a diagnosis of SLE or Systemic Lupus Erythematosus (lupus for short), was considered unusual in Britain. When I was told I had lupus, however, I was relieved that my condition had not been a figment of my imagination. I was told that it was a rare blood disease 'common to black females in the northern states of America'. I wondered how on earth I had got it.

I was 25 at the time, married with two young daughters. I live in Luton, Bedfordshire, in the South–East in Britain. Before I was diagnosed as having lupus, I worked as a secretary and I had hoped to take up nursing. After the diagnosis, I faced the prospect of 'pottering around' on steroid treatment for the rest of my life! Lupus is a disease of the immune system, which affects the connective tissues of the body, including blood. It can affect anyone, but is more likely to attack young women.

The disease affects nine women to every one man, and the incidence is higher in black people than white. Though in the past it was mainly found in women of childbearing age (20–45) modern diagnostic methods have found that it occurs in children as young as two, and in adults up to 90 years of age.

Lupus (which is Latin for wolf) is the name doctors in the past gave to various rashes on the cheeks and nose and is considered an ulcerated skin disease. Symptoms of lupus, which may occur singly or collectively, include allergy to sunlight; fatigue; skin rashes; fevers; joint pains; rheumatism; arthritis; hair loss; chronic circulatory problems; chest pains; pleurisy; kidney failure; cerebral involvement; strokes; and heart problems.

The disease is very debilitating, and symptoms displayed by patients may range from very mild to very severe. Lupus carries a heavy emotional and financial cost to the sufferer and to members of his or her family. These problems are increased by lack of understanding and sensitivity by members of the public, and more especially by members of professional bodies, including general practitioners, social services departments, nurses and policy-makers in statutory organisations.

Six years after my own diagnosis I met many white sufferers of lupus when I went to my first conference on the disease in London in 1979. I travelled with the mother of one white patient, whose daughter had been flung into a mental hospital, as had I, on a number of occasions. It made me realise that medics knew little about the disease.

At the conference I learned that in lupus patients make too many antibodies, which make us allergic to ourselves, and unable to fight infection. Possible causes of the disease were thought to be either: (1) genetic; (2) viral infection; (3) hormones; and (4) stress. There was no reference to black people, except for the presence of one black woman in a slide which was shown. There was no information about black people in the leaflets that were available.

Before the conference I had raised £400 for research into the disease. I was then asked to be the Bedfordshire contact on behalf of an arthritis organisation. I telephoned, wrote to or visited the twenty-five listed sufferers in my area and, faced with huge bills as a result, began to publicise and raise more funds. I displayed posters in libraries, doctors' surgeries, health centres and supermarkets. I held coffee mornings and jumble sales. Small amounts of money slowly began to come in from councils and local businesses.

Sometimes I booked a table in a local shopping centre. This gave me an opportunity to canvass the general public. I began to discover that lupus among whites was more common than I had been led to believe. I also learned that divorce and suicide rates were thought to be higher for lupus sufferers than for people with other disabilities. The work that I was doing had to be carried out between bouts of severe pain, acute depression, sickness and diarrhoea, and regular appointments to hospital for blood tests.

I visited people as often as I could; and felt comforted that I could relate to these new-found friends, rather than feeling isolated myself. Most of us were being treated with steroids and painkillers; some were taking stronger drugs for the pain, such as pethidine and morphine. Like me, some suffered with joint problems, depression and allergy to sunlight. Others complained of kidney, chest and/or skin involvement, among other things.

Looking back, I think my own health problems probably began when I caught a throat virus at the age of 14, while on a school trip to Holland and Belgium. I was treated with penicillin, after which my soprano voice dropped. I also had difficulty participating in sporting activities because of foot cramps. Period pains caused me to spend afternoons in bed with a hot-water bottle. I became anaemic. My throat was persistently sore, and in 1968, when I was 19, my tonsils had to be removed.

During the summer of 1969, my 8st. 3oz. weight

plummeted to 6 st. after a two-week bout of sickness and diarrhoea. I had no appetite and was so weak that I couldn't even sweep a room. I had to give up work as a temporary secretary. In all, my GP listed fourteen symptoms, including chronic hair loss and mouth ulcers, for my condition. I returned to work some weeks later, but kept falling asleep at the typewriter by 10 a.m. I managed to continue doing temporary work, with some difficulty. I was 20 at the time, and soon after I got married.

The following year a lump was removed from my right breast and I began to feel better. After the birth of my second child, however, I suffered with fevers, as I had done after the birth of my first child, when doctors had initially diagnosed me as having tuberculosis. After this, my monthly periods became erratic. I would feel ill one week before and after, leaving me just one week out of each month when I felt reasonable. My head was always heavy, but I just got on with life.

During the summer of 1972 I began to itch uncontrol-lably, and was prescribed drug after drug, to no avail. I writhed in agony after baths and became so fed up that I invited the local community relations officer to inspect my cupboard, which looked like a pharmacy! I just needed someone to believe that I was genuinely ill. The itching finally subsided after treatment with a steroid-based cream, prescribed by the hospital dermatologist. I asked for a referral to a London teaching hospital, because my throat problems persisted. Nodules were removed from my throat as a result, following which I attended speech therapy sessions until I was allowed to speak again.

A few weeks after this my wrist became painfully swollen, then my knees and ankles; and I noticed that my fingers were blue and painful, especially first thing in the morning. I burst into tears of frustration when I was told there was nothing wrong. I began itching again, and decided to change general practitioners after one threw a prescription at me.

I was admitted to hospital for tests, but extraction of two wisdom teeth prior to diagnosis caused heart, lung and kidney complications. I had been staying with my mother, who lived near to the hospital, when I had to be rushed in for treatment. My parents are strict and devout Christians, and my mother's only words, as I lay dying were: 'Pray Paula, Paula pray.' It was on this readmission to hospital that I was diagnosed as suffering from lupus.

I had to have oxygen, because I could barely breathe. My body was burning with fever. I was treated with 60mg of steroids daily, and I thought I would die every time the dosage was reduced. The paralysing chest and kidney pains took what seemed like an eternity to subside and I found myself thinking and acting outrageously after each dosage reduction. I was unable to walk for two weeks. I had to be lifted, turned, washed, dressed and fed by nurses for almost two weeks. I sweated so much during the night that nurses had to change the sheets at least once. I also suffered from vaginal thrush, which greatly distressed me.

When I was more able, I asked whether I might have passed something on to my elder daughter who in 1970 had also almost died. The doctor whom I'd asked (who happened to be black) turned on his heels and left, without replying. Upon my discharge from hospital I tried to find out why my teeth had been extracted, but again, no one seemed keen to answer.

When I returned home, we were given a home help, to allow me to rest. I had gained a lot of weight as a direct result of the steroid treatment, and I wanted to hide from the world. It was difficult to comprehend how much my life had changed, and I became very depressed, especially when I saw others enjoying life. My younger daughter was put into a day nursery, which really upset me, as I dearly wanted to care for her myself.

I slept all day when the family were out, and again in the evening, covered with a blanket on the sofa. I would then be awake all night. I was always cold, so cold that instead of wearing the fashionable clothes that I used to before my illness, I wore thick woollen ones. It was months before I could drive again. We were well supported by my parents, brothers and sisters. My suggestion for a family meeting to discuss my situation, however, was never taken up. My nerves were bad, and my confidence was gone. I even felt nervous about sewing and knitting, hobbies that had previously been natural talents. A visit to a cinema, after about six months, ended this spell of depression for a time.

My excessive use of the telephone, speaking to friends and relatives (because I felt so lonely), and central heating caused arguments with my husband, who had by now given up work to concentrate on writing for black publications. He constantly belittled my achievements, and when he moved out of our bedroom our marriage started to disintegrate. This was about 1979. I felt humiliated at having to apply for social security payments for myself and the children, because I come from a hardworking West Indian family.

I began to suffer with heavy nosebleeds and had twelve in one week. Again I was admitted to hospital, this time for a cauterisation. I felt dejected, but was befriended by members of a women's action group, which I had joined in 1974 – I was the only black member. Were it not for them and the assistance given by a good neighbour, my life would not have been worth living.

In the same year my husband had me admitted to a mental unit under a Section 25 Order, despite my protests that nothing was wrong with me. He believed I was acting irrationally, when I was in fact trying out naturopathic diets. On my release, I threw all the tranquillisers down the toilet and refused to speak to him.

I eventually divorced my husband in 1981, when I was 33, by which time I had had two hip replacements, tried to commit suicide, spent another spell in the mental unit and worked to repay our lapsed mortgage. I won an allowance for washing-up gloves because my fingernails had become infected. I also passed a German O-level examination, and began voluntary work with a health council. My mental state was seized upon by my husband in his successful court action to gain custody of my younger daughter. This hurt deeply, as the children had been my lifeline.

I was now responsible only for myself, as my older daughter had, by now, left home. I sang with a trad jazz band on alternate Sunday nights, and the phenomenal support I received from the musicians, the owner of the pub and the audience helped me regain confidence. In the same year, 1984, I won a mobility allowance,* after a battle which involved letters of support from my consultant, my MP and friends, and publicity in local newspapers. Knowledge gleaned from medics and other lupus sufferers prompted me to write a paper on the subject and led to involvement with a support group of which I became an active member.

In 1985 I was back in a London hospital, suffering from fluid in my lungs. I also eventually had a hysterectomy, because of heavy periods. More teeth were extracted from my deteriorating gums, and I could not stand being in the sun for more than a minute without feeling extremely sick. During this period I was constantly in and out of my GP's surgery with infections, bowel disorders, headaches and constantly painful joints.

I still suffered bouts of acute depression. I was not always able to walk, and had to spend a lot of time in bed. My shoulders became painful and I feared replacement operations, so I bought an automatic car which made driving easier. However, my mobility allowance was taken away, in

* Benefit that can be claimed from the Department of Social Security (DSS) on medical grounds, for those unable to walk due to physical disablement.

1987, after being renewed for just one year. Supportive letters from my MP and consultant made no difference. I appealed against the decision and was overjoyed when, in 1989, the mobility allowance was granted for thirty-five years!

Early on in my disease I had been consulting a rheumatologist at my local hospital in Luton, who remarked that I 'looked like the golly on a Robertson's jam jar!' After that, I asked for a referral to a London teaching hospital, where research was being carried out into lupus. It was the right decision. I learned that lupus was regarded as a 'dirty' disease, probably because lupus sufferers get so many infections and sweat from time to time because of fevers. My own experience bore this out to an extent – my body smelt rancid from drugs and sweats, my breath smelt too, and my urine stank. I learned that my fingers turned blue because I had what is known as Raynaud's disease, a condition brought on by cold and stress. My headaches were caused by inflammation of blood vessels in my brain. I also found out that this was a disease which baffled scientists.

In 1988 I was still working for a national arthritis organisation. I attended conferences, for example in Scotland, and made visits to lupus sufferers in my area, for which I received little financial assistance. Disillusioned with raising funds for an organisation that gave little support or respect when I most needed it, I decided to start my own lupus group.

Only two people – both black, and one a sufferer – were willing to form a committee. Membership of my new group increased rapidly, however, as sufferers from the previous group joined and I discovered other black sufferers in Luton. One woman was self-dialysising, because of a kidney complaint; and another could have died because of misinformation about the disease.

Also during this time, I was saddened to learn of the deaths of two other sufferers who lived locally, and who had become my friends over the years. I raised funds, held regular meetings and began to learn the intricacies of operating a charitable organisation. I am now in touch with lupus organisations in the United States, where there are said to be 500,000 sufferers. There is an exchange of information between my group and the Lupus Foundation of America (LFA) International Associates, sponsored by the Long Island/Queens Chapter. We receive up-to-date information from the LFA, but more work needs to be done on the disease in Britain.

Editor's note: The Luton & District Lupus Group, formed by Paula Thomas in 1989, aims to increase awareness of the disease and of the suffering it imposes or causes. The group provides support for sufferers and their families, as well as general advice on the disease to the public. It is a registered charity, with a membership of more than eighty.

Female Genital Mutilation and the Work of the London Black Women's Health Action Project

Shamis Dirir

I don't know where it comes from, but I think from the Egyptians. It's Somali women's culture, it's part of one's life.

The circumcision either makes you really angry or one becomes so passive that one continues in the role mapped out. It is another form of construction. Women are constructed for reproduction and man's pleasure. Her whole life is planned. From birth to death – it's settled.

(Extracts from *Silent Tears*, interviews on female circumcision)

ORIGINS OF FEMALE CIRCUMCISION

Female circumcision is practised in many parts of the world, mostly Africa and the Middle East, as well as some parts of Asia. In Europe the practice was thought to cure women suffering from nymphomania, hysteria, insanity or depression and was also used to correct clitoral hypertrophy (abnormal enlargement). It was a form of controlling resistance or potentially rebellious behaviour. The practice has recently re-emerged in America and in European countries, where a large number of immigrants from Africa and Asia have brought circumcision cultures from their countries of origin. In Africa, not one single country is spared this harmful practice. Some form of clitoridectomy or excision is practised in every country on the continent. Infibulation is mainly practised in Somalia, Sudan, Ethiopia, Mali and northern Nigeria.

Although female circumcision has apparently existed for centuries, no one knows exactly where or when it first appeared, nor what the underlying motives were. Some people believe that it has a religious basis, but the irony is that it is not practised in Saudi Arabia – the seat of Islam. It is not mentioned in the Koran, nor in the Old Testament (Hebrew Scriptures) or the New Testament. Male circumcision is mentioned in the first book of the Bible where it is stated that God ordered Abraham to circumcise his male children and all the other male children in the household.

Some scholars claim it originated around the Nile Valley during the Pharaonic era: young slave girls from the lower valley of the Nile were mutilated to curtail their sexual freedom and to reduce unwanted pregnancies. Female slaves in ancient Rome also had one or more rings put around the labia majora to prevent their becoming pregnant. Chastity belts were brought to Europe by Crusaders during the twelfth century.

Female circumcision is not practised by all Muslim nations. The practice is pre-Islamic, and reached the areas where it is currently entrenched before the spread of Islamic religion.

It is known that, in the history of mankind, many horrible things have been committed in the name of tradition, and taken for granted. As for circumcision, the primary reason for retaining the practice, in Somalia, Sudan and many other countries, is that it is a tradition. A Somali saying justifies the myth: 'The abandonment of a tradition annoys God.' For some tribes, circumcision is considered to confer eligibility for marriage. It is also claimed to be exclusively a women's affair, so mothers are obliged to make sure their daughters undergo this ordeal at the right time and in the most appropriate way.

WHAT IS FEMALE CIRCUMCISION?

Circumcision means the removal of the prepuce or hood of the female clitoris, or the foreskin of the male penis. The main difference between female and male circumcision is that in male circumcision no part of the sex organs is removed. The outer skin of the penis is cut without touching the penis itself.

There are three main types of female circumcision. They all involve serious health risks and have long-lasting effects on the lives of the women who undergo the operation; and yet there are no medical reasons for performing it. For this reason, it is felt that the term *female genital mutilation* (FGM) more fittingly describes the practice.

Sunna

This is the lesser form of FGM. It involves cutting off the prepuce or hood of the clitoris. In a sense, it is comparable to male circumcision, although sometimes a small cut is made on the tip of the clitoris to shed a few drops of blood. In other cases the tip of the clitoris itself is removed.

Excision (clitoridectomy)

A severe type of FGM, this involves total removal of the clitoris, the whole of the labia minora and the internal parts of the labia majora. (The labia minora cover and protect the opening of the vagina and the urinary opening.) After the healing process has taken place, a large scar forms to cover the upper part of the vulva region.

Infibulation

This is the most severe type of FGM. It involves total removal of the clitoris, the whole of the labia minora and internal parts of the labia majora. (The labia majora are the outer lips of the genitals which lubricate the inside of the skin folds to prevent soreness.) Afterwards, the two sides of the vulva are stitched together. A small opening is left at the lowest part of the vulva to allow the passage of urine and menstrual blood. This type of mutilation is called Pharaonic or Sudanese circumcision.

UNDER WHAT CONDITIONS IS FEMALE CIRCUMCISION PERFORMED?

In most cases, with the exception of those very few instances where the circumcision is carried out by a trained midwife or doctor, female circumcision is performed under very unhygienic and unsafe conditions, by an untrained, traditional midwife. Although there are some differences in the way the operation is performed, the damage done to the girl is always the same. That is the psychological harm, irrespective of whether a girl undergoes the mildest type of circumcision or is circumcised by a trained person.

At the time of the operation, the girl is held by at least three people – usually close relatives. One woman holds the girl's trunk and hands; while the other two women firmly hold her legs apart. The girl's buttocks are usually supported by a piece of wood. The circumciser sits or squats between the girl's legs and starts operating.

The instruments used for operation – generally unsterilised – include rough, traditional knives or razors. Besides the circumciser's ignorance of surgical techniques, the position she assumes while operating is so uncomfortable that unintended damage is almost unavoidable. This is because the site of the operation is such a considerable distance in front of her that she must stretch out to reach it.

Since the operation is performed without anaesthesia, the girl struggles and moves frequently, as do those who are holding her. This causes additional unintentional damage. In addition, a high rate of complications accompany female circumcisions. These can occur immediately after the operation or later on. They can be physical and psycho-sexual, minor or serious, even fatal in some cases.

MEDICAL COMPLICATIONS

Immediate complications

Shock
The pain of the operation, especially when performed without anaesthesia, to a child of 5–10 years who is fully awake, is so severe as to lead to shock. The clitoris and the labia are the most sensitive areas of the female body.

Bleeding
Bleeding is unavoidable. It occurs in all three types of circumcision, and is common in the sunna type because the dorsal artery of the clitoris is involved. The bleeding may be so severe that the life of the child is threatened if she is not transferred to a hospital for blood transfusion.

Infection
Infection is also inevitable, in view of the unhygienic way in which female circumcision is performed and the type of instruments used. Fatalities due to tetanus are known to occur.

Urinary complications
This condition is found in all three types of circumcision. It can arise either from the passing of urine in the raw area, from tight circumcision or as a result of an obliterated

orifice. In the latter cases, the child needs immediate relief. Acute urinary retention is a well-known complication that occurs within 48 hours of the operation.

Accidental damage to surrounding organs

This can occur as the result of a struggling child being operated on without anaesthesia. Injury has been reported to the urethra, anus and vagina. In some cases, injury to the vagina has ended in total occlusion (closure of the openings) and later the development of haematocolpos. This is a condition caused when the opening left for menstruation is too small; blood then collects and forms a bag-like mass in the vulva.

Long-term complications

Tight circumcision

This is a common complication, especially in relation to infibulation. The consequences of tight circumcision include difficult or impossible penetration, and pain during intercourse; difficulty in passing menstrual periods; difficult vaginal examinations including the inability to introduce a vaginal speculum during gynaecological examination or surgery; infection and injury to the vulva, due to repeated vigorous sexual acts which eventually lead to anal rupture.

Closure of the vaginal opening by scar tissue

This is due to the menstrual blood accumulating over many months in the vagina and urethra (haematocolpos).

Cysts and abscesses

Bartholin's secretions accumulate, forming cysts which later become infected and form abscesses on the vulva.

Keloid scars

The slow and incomplete healing of the wound and infection after the operation lead to the production of excessive connective tissue in the scar.

Difficulty in urinating

This is due to damage to the urethral opening at excision and infibulation.

Lack of cleanliness

Because of the difficulty in washing around the urethral opening, micro-organisms develop and ascend through the urethral opening, into the bladder. This leads to an inability to completely empty the bladder.

Prolonged and obstructed labour

This is caused by the tough and unyielding circumcision scar. It can lead to stillbirths, because of the prolonged and obstructed labour, and because of lack of oxygen in the vaginal canal.

LONDON BLACK WOMEN'S HEALTH ACTION PROJECT

The London Black Women's Health Action Project (LBWHAP) was set up in 1982 by a group of Somali and Arab women living or working in Tower Hamlets in London. Our focus was to develop a grassroots campaign to raise consciousness about and to eliminate the practice of female circumcision. Most of us who began the project were already working in black organisations in the area and were well connected in the communities. This was important, because we were under no illusions that we were tackling a difficult and contentious issue.

We took inspiration and courage from the fact that many similar campaigns are taking place in African countries which are committed to eradicating all forms of female genital mutilation. Little is known about the practice in Britain, however, and even less about the campaigns in Africa.

Those of us involved in starting the project were completely committed to two ideas. One was the complete eradication of the practice of female circumcision in all its forms, because we believe it is one specific aspect of the universal oppression of women. The other, related to strategy, was that we felt the best way to try and achieve this was at grassroots level, directly with women from the relevant communities, so as to begin to change their attitudes to the practice. We do this by supporting those members of the communities who demonstrate opposition to it. We have organised community-based workshops on the health dangers of the practice and exposed the fact that, contrary to much popular belief, the practice is not one which is prescribed in the Koran.

At the root of this strategy was the idea that a slower, more organic challenge to the practice was the way to achieve a permanent elimination of it. To begin the process and assess the extent to which there was concern within the communities, we carried out a three-month research project to find out about ideas and attitudes. The results confirmed the need to set up the project, working within the principles outlined above. LBWHAP became an unfunded voluntary organisation in 1982.

LBWHAP's work on female circumcision includes:

- casework with individuals, for example working with young women who are resisting pressure from members of the family for the operation to be performed; or work with mothers who are resisting pressure for the operation to be performed on their daughters;
- more general education and counselling on the harm and hazards of female circumcision;

- liaison with relevant statutory and non-statutory agencies on the effects of the practice; for example, by organising workshops and training sessions for community nurses and social workers;
- raising awareness within the communities and elsewhere about the legislation passed in 1985 which outlaws the practice of female circumcision in Britain, in all but a few circumstances; and
- direct work with schools and colleges.

LBWHAP has produced a book and video on female circumcision called *Silent Tears*. We have also produced a film with Channel 4, as well as numerous leaflets, posters and other materials, which are used in training and campaigning.

In response to demand, LBWHAP has also extended its work into other areas of health promotion within the black communities. We provide information and advice on sickle cell anaemia, as well as a general health information pack; and more recently we have carried out a pilot survey on the awareness of HIV and AIDs in the Somali community.

Though we have been able to obtain some funding from health authorities and other bodies, resources limit the extent to which the project can effectively expand its services or campaign on other health issues. This lack of resources has been keenly felt in recent months because of the rapidly increasing number of Somali refugees coming to London as a result of the war in Somalia. Not surprisingly, the new Somali refugee community, with its major material and emotional needs and lack of alternative support services, looks to the project as a potential source of support. In addition, because the new refugees often have counselling or physical health needs, professional agencies will often ask the project for advice and/or assistance to help meet the health needs of the new arrivals.

Since its small beginnings, LBWHAP has grown from an unfunded, grassroots black women's project into a well-established voluntary sector organisation in the community. We have developed links with a range of statutory and non-statutory professional agencies within health and personal social services.

INFORMATION, EDUCATION, COMMUNICATION

As our work has developed, an increasing focus has been the counselling of families as well as individuals about the specific issue of female genital mutilation and, in some cases, wider sexual problems. The more counselling the project offered, the more the need for such a service became apparent. However, we are unable, financially, to offer a fully fledged counselling service. Plus, simply to focus all of our attention on counselling would go against the overall campaigning aim of the project.

In an effort to resolve this tension, the project has given priority to community-based health education. Again, this is with a grassroots perspective, because we believe this is the best way to enable women in the community to develop confidence. They will then be better placed to understand their health needs and concerns, and this will increase the likelihood of the use of preventative health measures.

The need to run a series of health classes became a priority for the project. The first of these began in late 1987 and ran for one year. They were rotated throughout boroughs in north and east London, and were aimed at women affected by female genital mutilation. Their overall focus was women's reproductive systems in relation to circumcision.

CONSCIOUSNESS RAISING AND SUPPORT

Though the project is constrained in the amount of individual counselling it can offer, counselling still provides the axis around which the consciousness raising and campaigning aspects of LBWHAP's work is based. This is, of course, a common feature of many black and women's voluntary sector organisations. LBWHAP believes it can be most effective in stopping female circumcision by stimulating debate in the communities; debate which is framed in the cultural context within which the practice occurs. The project is clearly well placed to do this.

Three major aims underlie the approach which project workers take in counselling:

- to take a client-centred approach by supporting any decision to discontinue the practice of circumcision within an individual family;
- to raise consciousness about the health and legal implications of the practice of circumcision, in order that any actions are well-informed actions;
- to make every attempt to match the language and cultural background of counsellor and client.

ACHIEVEMENTS

The work with individuals and families, together with the health education classes, have proved to be vital in breaking down the taboos of talking about sexuality in general, and female circumcision in particular. As a result of LBWHAP's work, it is now increasingly possible to discuss these issues with women who were previously reluctant to do so, but who were most directly affected by the practice of female genital mutilation. Moreover, by questioning the very validity of female circumcision, the project is beginning to open up the whole field of male/female relations, making it subject to far-reaching discussions.

INTERNATIONAL CONTACTS

In keeping with the campaigning origins and focus of LBWHAP, we believe it is vitally important to keep up to date with international events and organisations that have relevance to the project's work. Members (workers and management committee) see themselves as part of an international feminist movement. Consequently, whenever possible, the project attempts to have representation at such venues. In 1985, for example, we sent a delegate to the International Seminar for Refugee Women, held in Holland. Our delegate led a workshop on the work being done in London. Later that year I attended the United Nations Women's Decade conference in Nairobi, which included a workshop on female circumcision.

The aim of attending such international events is to receive information, but also to publicise the work of the Project, and to establish the analytical, political and organisational links between work occurring in countries of origin, black communities in London and diaspora communities.

The central underpinning of the project remains its location as a grassroots women's organisation, with organic links to the communities from which it arose. Our future task is to maintain this base, as well as develop our feminist perspective on the issue of female circumcision, and of the wider issues related to women's health in general. As part of this effort we are planning a major international conference in May 1994, entitled 'Change Without Denigration'. Its aims are to put female genital mutilation on the world health agenda, with the fullest co-operation of the communities which practise it; to bring together groups, individuals and communities in Europe with an interest in female genital mutilation; and to share ideas and achievements and examine changes which have taken place in the past ten years in the NHS. In this way we hope to monitor progress and develop strategies that will encourage change in a sensitive and conscious manner; change which is acceptable to the communities who are directly affected.

A Career in the National Health Service: Making the Most of Equal Opportunity

Melba Wilson

Lynette Murray's career in the National Health Service has spanned thirty-three productive years. Entering the NHS as a student nurse in 1959, and retiring in 1992 as a director of Nursing and Midwifery Services in Wandsworth Health Authority, her career shows in microcosm the changes and developments in the health service, as they affect black people. Working through several reorganisations and at first seeing a drive towards equal opportunities for black people in the NHS, she now views with dismay and sadness the clawing back of the gains made; gains to which she, during her own career, was able to contribute. In one sense Lynette Murray's time in the health service chronicles the experiences of many black women who entered the service as nurses, in response to concerted trawls of former colonial countries by the British during the 1950s and 1960s. Black women were recruited to fill jobs in the service industries, which went begging amongst the indigenous population, jobs, for example, in the health service and transport.

In another sense Murray's experience is unique in that her rise through the ranks is not typical of the experience of most black people employed in the health service. More frequently they occupy low-paid, low-status positions in comparison to white workers, a situation that has remained unchanged. Murray's timing was to some extent fortunate: her decision to become a health service manager coincided with the NHS policy decision to pursue equal opportunities in employing black people. It is this, combined with Murray's refusal to take no for an answer, which accounts for her contributions to health care. Her achievements are measurable both in relation to the general population, and with regard to black people's health needs.

I first met Lynette Murray several years ago, when we both served on the management committee of a local community organisation working with black elderly people. Though I knew she worked in the health service, I did not know the wealth of experience and expertise she had as one of few black people who have 'made it' in the field, in the sense of receiving recognition for their work.

A few years later, while thinking about the structure of this chapter, I mentioned to a mutual friend that I was looking for a black woman to include because it was important to take note of the unique contribution of black nurses and other workers to the NHS. Lynette was suggested. She had just retired from the health service when we spoke, and was looking forward to starting a second career in another area of public service.

My hope, in helping to commit Lynette Murray's life in the NHS to record, is in part that it may inspire other black women and men who may view making such progress as an impossible task in today's less than opportunistic health service. I also feel it is important to provide a historical record of black people's achievements in every aspect of British life. Lynette Murray, one of the first black health service managers, deserves to have her career documented for those who follow, particularly given the shrinking numbers of those in similar positions.

Lynette was enthusiastic because, as she put it:

I think that black people ought to have the confidence to feel that they can get through. But the climate ought to be created within the government, within the [health] authorities, with those people who have the power to employ black people, to say: 'We will welcome you – provided you've got the qualifications and the right personality for the job – we will welcome you. We will train you.' The colour of your skin should not be the sole judge of whether you get the job or not.

Lynette Murray would be the first person to tell you that reaching the point that she did was not easy; that it required unswerving perseverance and a belief that she could achieve, despite all the obstacles. As a student nurse, almost immediately she had to contend with prejudice and low expectations. The place was Somerset, and the year 1959: the venue for beginning her nursing and midwifery training. For the 19-year-old Lynette, used to the warmth and hospitality of her native Guyana, arrival in a cold and racist Britain was a shock to the system.

When I got to Somerset, there were two other black girls there. The white people just weren't used to black people. When I walked down the road people used to say: 'Can I touch you so I can see what your skin is like?' When I spoke they said: 'I'm surprised that you can actually speak English. Where did you learn to speak English?' One of my fellow students even asked me if people like me lived in trees. At one point, I asked my mother to send a photograph of our house in Guyana, in order to give this girl the information she obviously needed.

Attitudes were no better among many of the hospital and teaching staff. Lynette remembers the unhelpful attitude of some tutors: 'There was a lot of prejudice among the tutors. If a black student got top marks that was completely ignored.' Added to this was the tendency of some white matrons to assign black students the more menial tasks on wards as a matter of routine. Lynette describes the form this took:

> We had to pass first-year exams and then go into second-year status. In your first year you did all the 'dirty' work on the ward, like cleaning bedpans, which we accepted as part of nursing. In second year, you were meant to move on to more sophisticated nursing – learning to do things like dressings. But we found that there were some sisters who always tried to put you down, and who wanted to keep you at the same level. There were two of us who were in the same set on one particular ward. The sister always made sure this particular girl [who was white] did the senior work and I didn't. I told the sister we were in the same set and I didn't think it was fair; but that I should get an opportunity to learn more senior work as well. She completely ignored me. I eventually went to the matron and complained. That changed things. When I went back to the ward this sister's attitude was quite different. She said to me that it wasn't meant; that she would make sure that I got the work done that I felt was entitled to me. I think she realised then that I wasn't someone she could mess around with.

Not surprisingly, the racism was not confined to staff and teachers. Some patients on the wards, for example, would refuse to have black nurses touch them. 'They were quite happy for you to take away their bedpans, but if it came to giving them injections or dressings, there were a few incidents where they didn't want it. They would call you names like blackie or blackbird,' said Lynette.

But she remained undeterred:

> I think coming from a place like Guyana helped. My father always used to say there is prejudice anywhere you go. Unfortunately, even in Guyana there was, because it was a colonial country. My father was a policeman. He used to say that if he saw a white person stealing, and he charged that white person, he himself would get into trouble. He always said the important thing was to make sure you had a good education and then you could fight your battles.

Coming to England therefore, I was more or less prepared for prejudice. But there were still some things which did hurt. But as time went on, one had black and white friends within the hospital, which was a supportive group. On our days off, we spent our time together, cooked for one another, shared our problems and gave each other advice, and gained strength from that.

The fighting of battles continued, however. Lynette completed her general training and qualified as a nurse in 1962.

When you are a qualified nurse you are in charge of the ward when the sister isn't there, so it's quite a responsible position. Despite that, you found some degree of prejudice. Because although you had a uniform to identify you as being a qualified person, some of the medical staff would come to the ward and look at you and look at the white student nurse, and go to her for information. Sometimes I used to say: 'Am I invisible?' That kind of thing happened a lot, not only to me, but to most black nurses I've met. I think it's the sort of thing that still happens, unfortunately. Although people can see there is a badge or a uniform, it's just as if one is invisible, and they just can't see you. But it makes you strong. You feel you've got to say something, so that people are aware that they are hurting you, and that it should be stopped.

Deciding that she wanted a career in midwifery, Lynette had to undertake further training – this time in Gloucestershire.

I applied to undertake midwifery training and went to Cheltenham. At that time we used to do Part One and Part Two midwifery, and you had a month in between while you waited for your exam results. In Cheltenham, they had a facility for some nurses to work for that month. That facility wasn't offered to the two black nurses there. So I decided to do some agency work. I went to the British Nurses Agency in Cheltenham. But they said: 'We don't employ people like you.' I said: 'What do you mean?' She said: 'We don't employ black people.' What hurt the most with Cheltenham was that they knew I was a foreign student, and they could have given me the facility of a month's work. But they didn't. There were English girls there who could have found jobs very easily, and they were offered that facility. Perhaps I didn't have the right accent.

The year was now 1963, and Lynette was forced to live on the savings she had managed to accumulate from her earnings as a student nurse. 'We didn't earn a lot of money. When I first started training, they provided a room, a uniform and food; and we earned £9 a month. Out of that £9, I used to send home £4 for my parents. So I was left with £5 a month, out of which had to come basics like tights and clothes.'

She survived that month with the help of friends and the comradeship of other black students. 'I found hostel accommodation in Bristol with the help of a friend. That was a safe place. It was cheap, because it was just a huge house with lots of rooms to let. I got a lot of support there because we were all black people and black students.' Next followed a stint in Birmingham, where she completed the specialised midwifery training. Birmingham also brought more and welcome contact with black people.

'Life was good. There were more black people; and there was a friendlier atmosphere because of it. You met more of your own people there. I used to go on the buses, and the conductor [usually black] would say: "I won't take fares from you," which was really quite nice.'

Successful completion of her training, which had involved working as a midwife in clinics and homes, brought a move to London. Marriage and the birth of Lynette's first child followed soon after. She then went to work on a part-time basis in Battersea General Hospital, as a nursing sister, but again, gaining the post meant surmounting another block: 'I had to fight for the sister's post, because the matron who offered me the job, was only willing to put me down as a staff nurse. It was only after I pointed out my qualifications and experience [six months as a staff nurse and one year as a midwife] that she offered me the post that was commensurate with my qualifications.'

In quick succession, Lynette moved on to become a district midwife and to continue training for clinical teaching. It was not easy to keep moving up the ladder:

I felt I needed to gain more clinical and teaching experience. But in order for me to do that in the health authority where I now worked, I had to do the training in my days off, because my boss said she could not give me the time off – even though being a clinical teacher would have helped not only me, but the organisation, in terms of giving me students to teach while I was a district midwife.

I finished the training and was, in fact, given two students – other midwives were given one. But it had been all on my own initiative. I got very little support from my managers. It was as a result of that and other experiences that when I became a manager, if I found staff who needed training, and who had the right push to want to get on, I would try and fight for them; for example, to allow them time off, and to get the organisation to pay for it.

In fact, I decided to go into management because of the frustrations that I felt at not being managed properly, and because of the problems that black people were having in the health service. I felt that maybe I could use my own experience and do a better job. At that time [1973], the health service was promoting equal opportunities for black people. I remember the first time I decided that I ought to try and see if I could get into management. I went to my first interview in Lewisham. I think it's always good practice for a manager, if they know that someone who's working with them is going for something completely new, to try to prepare them. But I had no preparation from my manager.

I went to the interview. They asked me about different reports that were out. I didn't know about a particular report. Afterwards, I went back and my boss asked me how I'd got on. I told her I didn't get the job because they had asked me about a report which I should have known about, but didn't. 'Oh,' she said, 'I could have told you about that.' So I asked to see a copy of the report. From then on I started preparing myself for interviews as if they were exams, and encouraged my peers to do the same. In August 1973 I got a job in Greenwich as a nursing officer. It was my first step into management.

Four years later Lynette obtained the job of senior nursing officer in Wandsworth Health Authority:

When I applied to Wandsworth, I felt I had a chance within the organisation because of the way the advert was written. Sometimes you can read from adverts who they're actually wanting to apply. And quite often you think, rightly, 'Oh well, that doesn't apply to me.' But the Wandsworth post asked for applications from all races, and I felt that did include me.

I was really surprised, though, when I was shortlisted and very pleasantly pleased. I was competing with an internal white candidate, and there were other white candidates as well. But I had obviously done a lot of work and that was recognised. In my interview for the job, they said they wanted black people who had something to offer. Having read my references, it was felt I was the person who could deal with challenges and problems as a black person. I soon found out why they felt that way. There were lots of problems at the hospital – problems to do with black staff in general. They didn't have anybody to speak up for them; and they felt there was a lot of unfairness in the way work was distributed, and the way they were treated – they weren't treated kindly. That was the legacy I inherited.

Lynette rose to the challenge – managing the services, instituting innovative practices, and at the same time, with care and understanding, also working to improve morale amongst black staff in her department. In part this was possible simply because she was a black woman in a hitherto unheard-of position of authority. Fortunately for her black staff, she was also a black woman who could and did take the time to empathise with her staff and their needs and concerns, in a manner which white colleagues had been unwilling or unable to do. Her reward, in addition to advancement in her career, was to receive the equally important approbation of black staff. 'They would come up to me and tell me how glad they were to see a black person in my position. They were proud.'

With rapid promotions came 12-hour days and hard work: 'I used to leave home at half-past seven and come back at half-past seven.' Promotion also brought Lynette the opportunity to institute change in her particular part of the health service.

> During the time I was at St George's, my department was able to achieve regional status in the neonatal field. The English National Board identified the midwifery and neonatal unit as one of the leading departments in the country. We humanised the service. That's because I'm a community person at heart. Having spent seven years as a district midwife, when my brain was ticking over with ideas, I felt I could use many of those ideas in the hospital.
>
> My department, for example, was chosen as one of the first to use link workers as advocates for patients who couldn't speak English. As a manager I could, and did, send one of our sisters on sickle cell and health education courses, so that she could advise people who came to the clinic. We also introduced community clinics in the health authority. In that way we brought the service to the people – doctors and midwives saw people in the clinics. When I left there were seven peripheral clinics. Before that, people were just herded; they came for appointments and waited and waited until they were seen.
>
> Before I left George's, I was looking at things like equal opportunities. I was monitoring recruitment and selection within the authority, because I felt that needed to be done if everyone, regardless of colour, was to have equal opportunity within that health authority.

Nevertheless, life at the top was at times isolating, despite the achievements:

> I was the only black manager there; and it's a very lonely job when you're at the top. Your staff may think you're a good manager. But I think that when you're at the top, you need somebody to say: 'How are you today?' You always have to present a happy or cheerful outlook, because that's the nature of the job. When you're in management, you've got to be a manager. You can't just say: 'Oh my God, where am I going to turn today?' You've got to have ideas and direction.

On the whole, however, says Lynette Murray, even accounting for the racism which appears to go with the territory of being black in a predominantly white society, hers was a smoother path than that currently available to black people wishing to pursue a career in health service management. Though she was able to make it through hard work ('which convinced them that they hadn't made a mistake'); and though she benefited from equal opportunity drives at a time when there seemed to be genuine good intent behind these, Lynette Murray feels that many young black women and men today have a much harder time even getting to first base.

> If you look at most health authorities now, there are very, very few black people in positions of authority. You'll find the porters and cleaners are black. You'll find the SENs [state enrolled nurses] are black. You'll find the nursing auxiliaries are black. But the thing that grieves me about the health authority now is that they're not identifying the bright, young black people who need to have an avenue to go ahead and get to the top. When I started with Wandsworth Health Authority in 1977, in my interview it was said they they felt they needed black people who had something to offer. They don't seem to want that any more.

Not only are young black people not being identified, but those who have gained a measure of success and recognition for doing a good job are slowly, but inexorably, losing ground, Lynette feels. 'Things seem to have gone backwards,' she said, in explaining what successive reorganisations of the health service have meant for black workers. She notes, for example, the trend now evident for many black people (some of them her former colleagues) who have held senior posts within health authorities, suddenly to find themselves 'reorganised out of a job'. 'One day a new structure comes out and you're not in it.'

Despite the seeming gloom, Murray remains optimistic. The spirit and resolve which saw her from those early, lonely days as a black newcomer to Britain through to becoming one of the first black NHS managers, continue to stand her in good stead for getting done what she feels it is still important and necessary to accomplish – equal opportunities for all. Now, however, her energies are being utilised by the voluntary sector.

> I do a lot of voluntary work, for example with the
> Maternity Alliance. I get the opportunity to go to Select
> Committees at the House of Commons. I give views on
> health services. I don't think I can get any higher than
> giving advice to the government, to tell them how we feel
> about things. I think you can tell them, when you have an
> opportunity, how you see they can make the best use of
> giving people an equal opportunity in providing a service.
> We also need to persuade our white colleagues as well; so
> that it's not only black voices calling for this. It should be
> something that everybody wants to happen.

But Lynette is under no illusions about the fact that black people pursuing careers in the health service, and in many other areas of public and private sector employment, face an uphill task. 'I don't know if it [equality of opportunity] will happen in my lifetime,' she said, 'but I like to think that my grandchildren will have an easier time. The secret is not to take no for an answer, and to have a positive approach to life.'

Early Motherhood and Black Women

Ann Phoenix

Has the last year as a mother been easy or difficult?

I think it's been easy and exciting really because she's talking now and she makes sentences and she asks to go places and that. Which is quite good.

(Single mother aged 18)

How would you describe him?

Oh, he's company. I really enjoy his company and I'm gonna miss that when I actually start going to work, but I really do enjoy that.

What do you enjoy about his company?

It's just being with him, really. I find that really sort of – absorbing, I should say.

(Single mother aged 16)

The above two quotes are from black mothers who gave birth in their teenage years and who, because of this, fit into a devalued age group of mothers which is the focus of a great deal of public concern. Both women were interviewed in a study of 16–19-year-old first-time mothers carried out at the Thomas Coram Research Unit at the University of London Institute of Education.[1]

These short extracts indicate that the two women got a great deal of pleasure from their children, who were then two years old. Yet, mothers under the age of 20 receive an almost universally bad press in both academic and more popular literature. Women who become pregnant in their teenage years are generally considered to have done so for reprehensible reasons such as because they have failed to use contraception correctly, or in order to get welfare benefits. They are also considered to be a 'drain on the state' once they have their children. For black women, in particular, 'teenage motherhood' is seen as one indicator of underclass status. It is also associated with poor educational attainment for both the mothers and their children, with complications of pregnancy and birth, and with child abuse. The concerns that can be picked out of academic literature and from the media are overlapping ones; the most frequently expressed is that women who give birth before they are 20 make inadequate parents.

The issue of teenage motherhood also provides a clear example of how negative perceptions about black people in general are produced and perpetuated. For while 'teenage motherhood' is stigmatised in both the US and in Britain, concern is expressed more frequently and is often more heightened about black 'teenage mothers' than about their white peers. Indeed 'teenage/adolescent/young motherhood' has often been considered a 'black problem'.

Public concern about single black teenage mothers in the US developed in a context in which black family structures had already been defined as problematic by some writers:

> The point implied in much of the literature is that a lot of the culturally 'abnormal' behaviour of minority groups can be traced back to supposed family deficiencies. Additionally, the problematic black family background is often implicated in explanations for unrest, decay and violence in the inner cities.[2]

> The intellectual history of this problem [lone black mothers under 20] begins not with teenage pregnancy, which only became a public concern around 1970, but with worries about black family structure that began in the 1960s with the Moynihan Report (1965).[3]

In societies where black family structures are held responsible for producing inner city problems of poverty and crime, the identification of an association between blackness and another stigmatised family grouping ('teenage mothers') produces moral panic. The children of single black mothers are widely viewed as problematic for society; and they and their mothers are regarded as little more than a drain on the state's resources.

Most Western societies are concerned to influence the quantity and quality of children produced.[4] Societies such as those of Britain and the US are permeated by racial discrimination and racist ideologies against blacks and other minority groups. As a result, fears about 'race' and reproduction focus more public attention on devalued groups of black mothers than on similar white groups and make them a potent political issue. Thus while black mothers and children are frequently omitted from research studies when 'normal families' are being studied there are many studies which focus exclusively or predominantly on black, lone and/or teenage mothers.[5]

Martha Ward interviewed professionals working in the field of 'adolescent pregnancy' in Louisiana. She suggests that the thinking of black and white professionals about adolescent pregnancy, is different:

> Many leading black professionals state their views that population policy, certain economic policies, and programs for adolescent pregnancy are, in fact, a 'hidden white agenda'. In private interviews, the fears of genocide are openly discussed . . . At the regular conferences and task force meetings held on the subject, white leaders will go to

elaborate lengths to dissuade their black colleagues that genocide is not the population policy of either the U.S. government or the state of Louisiana.

The white social-structural model is built on the ideal of 'the quality of urban life.' At the conservative end of the spectrum, the concrete concerns are crime, the cycle of poverty, or the availability of trained and willing workers . . . The liberal end of the spectrum will emphasize the rates of infant mortality . . . good prenatal care and the now voluminous documentation about the relationships of age at first pregnancy, family size, educational achievement, career development and social mobility.[6]

The arguments presented in this chapter do not assume that early motherhood is necessarily a problem and that it is worse for black than for white mothers under the age of 20. The starting point is a consideration of whether early motherhood is as problematic as much academic and popular literature suggests. I will discuss ways in which a focus on black women in considerations of 'teenage motherhood' obscures an understanding of early motherhood. Finally, I look at the health implications of early motherhood for black women.

My arguments are that 'teenage motherhood' is not cause for generalised concern, and that it is unsatisfactory to assume (rather than to establish) causative and outcome differences, between mothers under 20 who are from minority groups, and those who are white. In discussing these arguments I will consider the interrelationship of early motherhood and poverty. This is because debates on the 'feminisation of poverty' and on the emergence of an 'underclass' in the US, and renewed interest in poverty and its effects in Britain, have fuelled concern that 'adolescent parenting' causes poor economic outcomes for women and children.

Given such concerns, the question of whether mothers under 20 do make bad mothers is obviously a relevant one.

DO MOTHERS UNDER 20 MAKE INADEQUATE MOTHERS?

There has been an enormous outpouring of research literature on mothers under 20. Almost all of it concludes that motherhood in this age group presents problems. Yet, perhaps surprisingly, there is no clear evidence that with regard to social and developmental outcomes mothers aged under 20 and their children really do fare badly.

> Some researchers suggest that the evidence on which the worrying conclusions described above have been based is rather weak and that the negative aspects of early motherhood have been overstated.[7]

> More recent studies which control for such factors as SES [socioeconomic status], nutrition . . . and so on . . . reveal good obstetric and paediatric outcomes among adolescent mothers.[8]

Far from being inadequate mothers, most of the young women in the study carried out at the Thomas Coram Research Unit, were caring well for their children. They reported that they loved their children and got a great deal of satisfaction from motherhood. These findings – together with work that is critical of literature which stresses the negative consequences of early motherhood – indicate that most mothers under 20 are not inadequate. It was clear from their accounts that the vast majority of the women (both black and white) in the Thomas Coram study were far from being inadequate mothers: they chose to put time into doing things with their children and observed their children's behaviour affectionately:

> If [she's] awake I sort of like teach her little things, like how to count. 'Cos she can count up to ten now, and say a *little* bit of her ABC, except when you say 'A', she jumps to 'D', and um play with her little games like ring a ring o' roses and all that lot. (Mother of two-year-old daughter, aged 16)

He's very boisterous. Mischief! On the whole he's a really good boy. He is. A great little imitator. He loves to imitate, as you know! . . .

Would you say that it's easy or difficult looking after him?

Easy. No way is he difficult. (Mother aged 17)

It may be believed, since the mothers in this study were young women, that they merely had an intuitive grasp of what they should do with their children. However, most demonstrated theoretical knowledge when asked directly about the sorts of things that helped children to be healthy and happy. They were clearly aware of the current state of knowledge about how to encourage children's development:

What do you think affects the way that children grow up?

I think it's the atmosphere they're brought up in, really. I suppose it could be in their genes, but I think it's the atmosphere they're brought up in. That's what does it, really.

What about so the child grows up happy?

Just to make him happy. Like if you've got family arguments try and keep it away from the child. Don't argue in front of him and fight – don't do it at all, but if you have to, don't do it in front of the kids.

What about so that he grows up healthy?

Give him all the fresh food, vitamins he needs. (Mother aged 19)

FAILING TO FIT NORMATIVE ASSUMPTIONS

If poor outcomes (i.e., inadequate mothering, leading to inadequate childhood development) do not account for the negative reports on motherhood in the under-20s, we need to find other explanations. A major reason is that these young women fail to conform to current social expectations about what 'good mothers' *should* be like. This section discusses five normative assumptions that most mothers under 20 fail to fit at the time they give birth.

Moral reasons

'Good mothers' are supposed to be married before they conceive. Yet nowadays 80 per cent of mothers under 20 in Britian are single when they give birth. It is true that an increasing number of births in all age groups are now registered as being to women who are not legally married, but those under 20 are more likely than any other age group to be single when they give birth. The next highest rate of births to single women is to those in the 20–24 age group, almost a quarter of whom are single when they give birth. 'Teenage mothers' do not, therefore, conform to dominant reproductive ideologies which prescribe that marriage should precede conception. Mothers of this age appear to pose more of a threat to the institution of marriage than do older mothers, and when the decline of the family is being discussed, 'teenage mothers' are generally singled out for negative attention. In such discussions the lack of contribution that unemployed or low-paid men can make to women and children is rarely considered. Yet, in the Thomas Coram study it was clear that women were more likely to marry if their male partners could make some financial contribution to their households.

It is also true that a higher proportion of pregnancies is terminated in the under-20 age group than in any other (nearly a half in the US and nearly a third in Britain, with a greater proportion of the relatively few under-16s who become pregnant having abortions). Partly as a result of the availability of legal abortion, motherhood is now less common in the under-20 age group than it was three decades ago.

Currently no British data are available on rates of marriage, early motherhood and abortion for black women, yet it is widely assumed that black mothers are more likely than are white mothers to be single parents.[9] Evidence from the USA does indicate that black teenage women are more likely than their white peers to be single when they give birth. But in fact the difference is diminishing, because the rate of births to young single white women has increased dramatically in the last decade. Nonetheless, black mothers frequently appear in published work only as the heads of 'female-headed households'. The rationale seems to be that they are the only group of women to which the term 'female-headed households' applies; and that they are unlikely to live in any other family form. It is perhaps not surprising then that black mothers under 20 are considered more problematic than white ones. However, evidence from the USA suggests that marriage is not particularly desirable for young black women who become mothers:

> For whites, marriage operates as a major recovery route, offering an alternative or, at least, an important supplement to their own earning ability. Low education and restricted job opportunities, therefore, are not quite as costly as they are for black young mothers. On the other hand, the advantages of delaying parenthood are not so great for blacks as well . . . The cruel fact is that for blacks delaying childbearing has a relatively low payoff. They are damned if they do and damned if they don't.[10]

Furstenberg *et al.*'s seventeen-year longitudinal follow-up of black mothers who had been 17 years old when they had their first child similarly found that marriage did not help most young black women financially:

We also must report that marriage per se contributes little to a woman's economic chances . . . Only those who married early and remained married escaped economic disadvantage, and . . . many of the early marriages quickly dissolved.[11]

Many black women and white women in the Thomas Coram study had negative feelings about marriage and felt that they themselves would not wish to marry:

The majority of people I know haven't got nothing out of it [marriage] . . . To me I could never get married because I've sat down and watched my mum and dad's marriage fall apart and I wouldn't like to go through that myself. I mean they [men] come home, find the kitchen clean, food waiting . . . They get a little slave. (16-year-old single woman in pregnancy)

I mean I've always been told that a man's meant to be faithful to you if you're married and that . . . I feel sorry for some of these women who are married and then their husband's – he's no good and that, and I don't think it's any better for women who are married. I think it's just luck if you stay together. (19-year-old woman; cohabiting)

Concerns about state dependence

Many mothers in this age group in Britain and the US are dependent on state provision of housing, and on income support. Since part of the social construction of good parents is that they should make independent provision for their children, this makes them subject to public censure. For some, it also confirms the underclass status of mothers under 20. There has been much speculation that young women become pregnant in order to get housing and welfare benefits, but studies that have investigated this motivation have found no confirming evidence. Nonetheless there is, in some quarters, disapproval of such women's reliance on state benefit, which many people assume is a direct effect of childbearing and childrearing. Such dependence is, however, the result of the young women's educational and employment histories, and of those of the men who father their children. Women who give birth before they are 20 generally have few educational qualifications and find it difficult to find permanent, well-paid jobs. They have generally already experienced poverty and poor employment before conception.

In the Thomas Coram study only 20 per cent of the 16–19-year-old first-time mothers interviewed had one O level or equivalent (national exams which, like the General Certificate of School Education which replaced them, were generally taken at 16 years of age in Britain). Many had experienced periods of unemployment before they became pregnant, as had their children's fathers. Their parents had also suffered higher than average rates of unemployment. For many women, there was no evidence that either deferring motherhood or marrying would necessarily lead to an improvement in their economic circumstances. Indeed, many mothers who are over 20 years of age when they give birth also live in poverty. It was partly because of this that some women felt that they had no reason to defer motherhood beyond the teenage years. However, poverty, intertwined with dependence on welfare benefits and council benefits, was, for many of the young women in the study, the greatest problem they faced:

I mean sometimes I've had lots of bills to pay and I've had to pay the bills and gone without.

What have you gone without?

Oh food. Mostly food. Sometimes we had to go round my mum's or dad's to get some food because there's nothing here to eat.

But you managed to pay the bills?

No, they did cut me off [electricity]. Even though they weren't supposed to they still came . . . So the DHSS had to get in touch with them and hassle them to put it back on. (Mother aged 18)

What Social Security is giving me I really have to struggle on it. And most of the time I'm always broke until the next money comes in but I just do without until the next money comes in. (Mother aged 19)

It's like I really have to beg them for somewhere to live and . . . you know, that's bad. (Mother aged 19)

Elaine McCrate argues that black women who become mothers in their teenage years anticipate accurately the discrimination they will face in the employment market.[12] As a result, they have less incentive than do white women to avoid teenage births and these are not as economically costly for black as for white teenagers.

Since both underclass status and dependence on state benefits are associated with black populations in the USA and in Britain,[13] the intersection of two negative social constructions ('young mothers' and black people) is detrimental to the social construction of black mothers under 20.

Unplanned, unwanted and uncared-for children

Reports that mothers aged under 20 tend to have unplanned pregnancies have generated the concern that children are not really wanted. This runs counter to the notion that parenthood should be prepared for. Studies generally find that only between a quarter and a third of teenagers who conceive have 'planned their pregnancies'. The Thomas Coram study found that teenage women had not become pregnant because they lacked the necessary knowledge of contraception. They had become pregnant for a range of reasons. Some had decided that they wanted to have a child.

Were you trying to get pregnant?

Yes . . . When I used to work in the nursery I used to take like three children home on my weekends . . . and he loves kids as well, so we used to . . . babysit for 'em – play mummy and daddy sort of thing, and then we decided it would be best if we had our own instead of taking other people's kids, 'cos I used to feel a bit sad you know when I had to bring 'em back. So we decided to have our own. (Woman aged 19)

The study also found that some of the women who did not claim to have 'planned their pregnancies' actually did not mind whether or not they became pregnant because pregnancy and childrearing would not be a particular disruption of their lives or employment prospects:

It wasn't really bothering me if it happened. I always knew I'd have support from my family. (Mother aged 19)

Were you trying to get pregnant?

Yes I sort of planned it . . . I was thinking that if I do – I'm not definitely going out of my way to get pregnant, but if I do get pregnant, well, I'm happy and I'm keeping it because I love kids and I couldn't see myself waiting until I'd eventually settled down and that because it seemed a long way off . . . because I seemed to be having it difficult by not finding jobs easily like I used to before and, you know, everything. So I was thinking I might as well get settled down now. (Mother aged 19)

Even women who had considered it important not to become pregnant were delighted to be having a child by the end of pregnancy. Their intentions beforehand did not always influence their feelings afterwards: 'And I'm really looking forward to it, you know. I've come to terms with it. It's taken a long time, but . . . ' (18-year-old woman).

Despite the lack of well-founded evidence, concerns persist that mothers under 20 make inadequate mothers whose children are themselves likely to become social problems. This parallels the ways in which black parents have been labelled as inadequate to the task of rearing children who achieve reasonable educational qualifications and are not delinquent.[14]

Are adolescents mature enough to be mothers?

The period of adolescence is regarded as the time which links childhood and adulthood but is neither. It is, however, difficult to be certain when adulthood has been reached, particularly since the attainment of legal rights and responsibilities occurs at different ages.

The boundaries between childhood and adulthood have become less well defined over the course of this century. Longer compulsory education and increasing participation in further education have kept more teenagers in a dependent status for longer. The high rate of youth unemployment means that fewer young men from low-status socioeconomic groups are able to signal their transition to adult status by obtaining their first pay packet. The marriage rate for teenage women has also declined. The signifiers of adult status are thus unlikely to be gained in the teenage years. They are, arguably, harder for black than for white young people to achieve because racial discrimination produces a higher rate of black than of white youth unemployment. In addition black young people tend to stay longer in full-time education than do their white peers.

The status of 'adolescent mothers' is even more ambiguous than that of teenagers in general, because they are perceived as having taken on adult responsibilities during a period in their life when they are not regarded as adult. Yet the majority of women who give birth before they are 20 are actually 18 or 19 years of age. It is debatable whether most can really be considered adolescent.

Women from devalued groups are most likely to become 'teenage mothers'

It is well established that women who become mothers in their teenage years tend to come from families that are larger than average, to have parents who are more likely to have divorced and more likely to be dependent on welfare. The men who father their children come from similar backgrounds.

In the USA, as we saw earlier, black women are more likely than white women to become mothers in their teenage years. Although British figures are not available, it has been suggested that a similar disproportion exists. Some local studies suggest that there is a higher incidence of early motherhood among 'West Indian' women, and that West Indian women are more likely than white women to remain single when they give birth in their teenage years.[15] Yet there is little systematic evidence for this. A representative national survey of mothers in their teenage years found that 4 per cent were 'West Indian' and 5 per cent were Asian.[16] This may not be an over-representation of young black women in the under-20 age group since in some areas young black people constitute a higher proportion of their age group than older people do. Until national figures are available it is impossible to be sure of the incidence of early motherhood among black women. However, since eighty per cent of all women who give birth in their teenage years are single at the time when they give birth, and the population of young black women of African-Caribbean descent constitutes less than the 3 per cent of all British young women under 20, it is unlikely that the relatively few black British women of African-Caribbean origin could be responsible for the national rates of single motherhood.

The fact that women from socially disadvantaged backgrounds are more likely to give birth in their teenage years confirms many people's views that early motherhood is problematic and undesirable.

By virtue of their social class and often their colour and gender (white and middle class), researchers and journalists are usually socially distant from the young women about whom they write. A problem-centred approach to early motherhood is easily produced and reproduced by them. Professionals who work with 'young mothers' expect to find problems and therefore stress negative findings, even if only a minority of 'young mothers' are found to have problems.

HEALTH IMPLICATIONS FOR BLACK WOMEN

Most young women (both black and white) who give birth fare well. Nevertheless, a consideration of the health implications of early motherhood for black young women needs to be focused on ways to foster good outcome and alleviate any poor outcomes for the women and their children. It is clear from the Thomas Coram study that social support is crucial. Emotional, financial, childcare and other practical types of support all have an important part to play. Women's friends and families and, if available and supportive, their children's fathers, can all contribute to a good outcome. Indeed, the women's mothers were found to be particularly supportive. The following black young woman, asked if there is anyone she could leave her daughter with while she went out, replied that her parents would always look after her daughter and that, 'It's like putting gold in their laps.'

In the following instance, the woman speaking left her cohabitee and moved back to her mother's house with her baby because she found life easier there:

... I mean my sisters they're better mothers than I am ...
They're excellent. I mean – I think if it wasn't for them two
I'd've really been stuck. (Mother aged 16)

Mothers were often as economically supportive of their
daughters (and grandchildren) as they could be. This sometimes took the form of provision of free or extremely cheap
board and lodging:

I decided to tell my mum that I wanted to give her money
for food ... So she said to me that I don't have to pay.
And I don't really have to give money for food. But because
I'm staying here I'm going to want to eat more and she can't
really afford it. (Mother aged 19)

The high rate of single motherhood among mothers under
20 should not be disapproved of in a mechanical manner. In
the Thomas Coram study, many male partners did not provide much support, of any kind and marriage was more
likely for women whose male partners were able to make an
economic contribution to the women and their children.

The availability of adequate welfare benefits and council
housing are important, given the high rate of employment
for young people and the fact that almost all young women
who give birth in their teenage years come from sections
of the working class which have high rates of dependence
on such payments and housing.

Adequate provision of access courses (preferably with
crèche facilities) for black women returning to study are
also important. For a few women in the Thomas Coram
study, having a child actually gave them the impetus to gain
educational qualifications or to seek training so that they
could show their children that it is possible to achieve
educationally, and so that they could give them a better
standard of living. This may be especially important to
black young women because, in British society, young

black people of African Caribbean origin tend to gain few educational qualifications at school.[17] However, their commitment to education is such that many stay on longer in further education than their white peers in order to gain initial qualifications.

CONCLUSIONS

Many studies of mothers under 20 find that 'teenage motherhood' is not a widespread social problem. Instead it is a minority of 'young mothers' and their children who fare badly. The concern early motherhood evokes is partly because negative outcomes are generally highlighted in research reports, but it is also the result of an interrelationship between moral concerns, ambivalence about the nature of adolescence, concerns about high levels of state dependence in 'teenage mothers' and the social distance between young women who become mothers under 20 and the professionals and researchers who study them. This raises the question of whether most of those who write on early motherhood are implicitly assuming that behaviour that is well suited to white middle-class lifestyles would also be suitable for mothers under 20 (few of whom are from the middle class).

The major problem that mothers of this age group face is economic, but early childbearing is not the cause of poverty. Low socioeconomic status usually pre-dates pregnancy and motherhood for these women. There is currently little conclusive evidence about whether some mothers under 20 would fare better if they deferred motherhood. Early motherhood may well be a positive strategy for young women who have few opportunities for employment advancement. This is because they have their children before poverty has taken as great a physical toll on them as it is later likely to,[18] and they do not have to forego the earnings that women in more privileged positions often have to.[19]

A good understanding of 'teenage motherhood' cannot be fostered by the simple assumption that black mothers and white mothers are culturally different. The interpretation of the little that we know about black/white differences in reproductive patterns that have been recorded requires recognition of commonalities in black women's and white women's reasons for becoming mothers early in their life course, and for remaining single when they do so. These commonalities are related to structural factors such as higher rates of unemployment. Such factors economically disadvantage black people in comparison with white people and hence influence different patterns of behaviour. But stereotypes of black mothers under 20 as either more or less problematic than white mothers under 20, and as having either more or less supportive parents, are inaccurate and outdated.

Notes

1. This research project is written up more fully in Ann Phoenix, *Young Mothers?*, Cambridge, Polity, 1991. All the women whose words are quoted in this chapter are black. The age given is their age at the time when they gave birth.
2. Arthur Brittan and Mary Maynard, *Sexism, Racism and Oppression*, Oxford, Basil Blackwell, 1984, p. 134.
3. Constance Willard Williams, *Black Teenage Mothers: Pregnancy and Childrearing from their Perspective*, Lexington, Mass., Lexington Books, 1990, p. 1.
4. See Ann Phoenix, 'Black Women and the Maternity Services', in J. Garcia, R. Kilpatrick and M. Richards (eds), *The Politics of Maternity Care: Services for Childbearing Women in Twentieth Century Britain*, Oxford, Clarendon Press, 1990.
5. See Ann Phoenix, 'Narrow Definitions of Culture: the Case of Early Motherhood', in S. Westwood and P. Bhachu (eds), *Enterprising Women: Ethnicity, Economy and Gender Relations*, London, Routledge, 1988.
6. Martha Ward, 'The Politics of Adolescent Pregnancy: Turf and Teens in Louisiana', in W. Penn Handwerker (ed.), *Births and Power: Social Change and the Politics of Reproduction*, San Francisco, Boulder Press, 1989, pp. 151–2.

7. Frank Furstenberg, Jeanne Brooks-Gunn and S. Philip Morgan, *Adolescent Mothers in Later Life*, Cambridge, Cambridge University Press, 1987.

8. Dimity Carlson, Richard La Barba, Joseph Sclafani and Clint Bowers, 'Cognitive and Motor Development in Infants of Adolescent Mothers: A Longitudinal Analysis', *International Journal of Behavioral Development*, 9 (1) (1986): 1–14.

9. See Ann Phoenix, 'Narrow Definitions of Culture'; and 'Black Women and the Maternity Services'.

10. Frank Furstenberg, 'Race Differences in Teenage Sexuality, Pregnancy, and Adolescent Childbearing', *Milbank Quarterly*, 65 (1987): 381–403; quote from pp. 396–7.

11. Furstenberg *et al.*, *Adolescent Mothers in Later Life*, p 67.

12. Elaine McCrate, 'Discrimination, Returns to Education and Teenage Childbearing', paper presented to the Middlebury Conference on Discrimination Policies and Research in the post-Reagan Era, 6–8 April 1989.

13. William Julius Wilson, *The Truly Disadvantaged: The Inner City, The Underclass and Public Policy*, Chicago, University of Chicago Press, 1987.

14. See Errol Lawrence's chapter in Centre for Contemporary Cultural Studies *The Empire Strikes Back: Race and Racism in 70s Britain*, London, Hutchinson, 1982; and Paul Gilroy, *There Ain't No Black in the Union Jack*, London, Hutchinson, 1987.

15. See Carolynne Skinner, *The Elusive Mr Right*, London: Carolina Publications, 1986.

16. See Madeleine Simms and Christopher Smith, *Teenage Mothers and their Partners*, London, HMSO, 1986.

17. See, for example, The Swann Report, *Education for All*, London, HMSO, 1985; and Richard Skellington *'Race' in Britain*, London, Sage, 1992.

18. Arline T. Geronimus, 'On Teenage Childbearing and Neonatal Mortality in the States', *Population and Development Review*, 13 (1987): 245–78.

19. Heather Joshi, 'The Cost of Caring', in C. Glendinning and J. Millar (eds), *Women and Poverty in Britain*, Brighton, Wheatsheaf, 1987.

The Lambeth Women and Children's Health Project: Working With Child Sexual Assault

Patricia Joy Agana

> Nobody
>
> Nobody could touch me.
> Nobody was allowed to.
> Then why had he placed his hand there?
> Was he allowed to because he was nobody? Was he? . . .
>
> Nobody hurts us.
> We don't like nobody.
> Nobody likes us.
>
> Brenda Hayde–Agard[1]

Lambeth Women and Children's Health Project is an organisation primarily concerned with the health and welfare of women and children. We are a community health project, and work with childhood sexual assault currently makes up one third of the work that we do; the other two-thirds is concerned with HIV, pregnancy testing, parenting and other generic women's health issues.

Alongside the development of feminism were always Black women. Some were desperately trying to be accepted by this great new social consciousness. Others noted its failings with respect to race, and created an alternative forum, where Black women could have space to go through a process similar to that of the feminist movement without, overtly at least, being hindered by the negative dynamics of racial oppression.

Black Power had been the precursor of all the liberation movements yet there was no acknowledgement of the contribution that women of African, Asian and Caribbean[2] descent could make to the feminist debate. The myths about African peoples, and in particular our sexual behaviour, are a legacy of slavery. The myths were designed to justify the rape and the abuse of African women, who were used as breeders to supply a labour force for the plantations. Historically, we were described as 'sultry' or 'seductive', and as having 'hidden mysteries' and an 'animal charm'. Indeed, we continue to be described this way by popular newspapers and fashion magazines. This mythology erroneously informs professional and lay people alike in their understanding of child sexual assault within African and Asian communities.

Despite the direction of the feminist movement, it too, was conditioned by the sexual mythology surrounding Black women. At best, the movement's underlying perceptions of Black women contained derogatory racial misconceptions; at worst we were written out of history. Even the new-found energy of the white lesbian movement had room for Black women only in the bedroom, on the dance floor, or as personal trophies of their own political correctness. It was against this background that women of African, Caribbean and Asian descent met to discuss and support women who had experienced and suffered childhood sexual assault in their lives.

We met in Black women's centres. The Brixton Black Women's Centre was the first in the United Kingdom, and I was fortunate enough to be working there while I was a student; I ran summer projects for Black children. I also used the centre as a haven, a place of solace – somewhere to go and think, to rest, to badger staff with questions about the meaning of life, love, relationships, the role of Black women and our future.

Marlene Bogle was a central figure in the Black Women's Centre, setting the tone of the place. Sometimes we would talk about being Black Women. At other times women would come to her and she would disappear, with an official air. There would be silence, a secrecy that I did not understand. Another woman who made an impression on me was Chris Black, a young black feminist who had been involved in making documentaries about incest and child-hood sexual assault, as well as campaigning for the voice of survivors to be heard. It was not until some time later, when Marlene and Chris held the first national conference for Black women survivors of childhood sexual assault and went on to form a support group for Black women, that it became clear to me that for some years Marlene had been counselling Black women who had suffered childhood sexual assault. She was the first Black woman I had met who was working in this area, at that time a very lonely position for a Black woman. It was under her guidance that Lambeth Women and Children's Health Project decided to research and develop services in this area.

In 1986 I was invited by the project's management committee to carry out research into childhood sexual assault. At that time, vast strides were being made in the field by the feminist movement. Women who had suffered sexual assault identified themselves as survivors, a political concept intended to overturn the persistent powerlessness implied by the term 'victim'.

My work with the project required me to attend meetings, seminars and conferences, as well as to interview different individuals and organisations: Lambeth Women and Children's Health Project works for all disadvantaged women and children. As a Black woman, I bring to the work the benefit of my perceptions, and I was constantly being approached by women who had been sexually assaulted. I quickly became aware that it was not appropriate to raise such trauma in people's minds without providing some means by which they might be heard, or some way for them to resolve their feelings. To enable me to do this I trained as a counsellor with the London Rape Counselling and Research Project (LRCRP). I then went on to facilitate workshops and run training courses for social services departments, taking care to ensure that this work was informed by my practice as a counsellor.

My work gave rise to enquiries from professionals about the management of cases involving Black families, and the particular difficulties encountered by Black professionals in the field in working with white families and white colleagues. Race had then begun to rear its head as a complicating factor in the many approaches to working with sexual assault. A significant number of calls came from outside Lambeth from professionals who, because of limited resources and a lack of information, were unable to make informed decisions. Counselling agencies were also referring Black women on to us.

In 1989 the work generated by my investigations became overwhelming. In an effort to move from simply collecting information to delivering an effective service it became necessary to 'cut our coat to match our cloth'. The project then had only one worker in this area, and that was myself. The focus became one-to-one counselling and training for institutions. At this stage the main service users were white women with sufficient social awareness and feminist political history to understand the benefits of counselling. Black women were not to make extensive use of our service for a further two years. I had trained and worked with the London Rape Counselling and Research Project in preparation for the delivery of a counselling service; throwing out the negatives of that experience and developing the positives to ensure that we provided counselling which respected all cultures, all races and social norms. The experience with LRCRP more than prepared me for the onslaught that was to follow.

Researchers appeared at our door wanting information about the incidence and prevalence of child sexual assault in Black communities. So did we!!! But this information did not – and still does not – exist in any co-ordinated form. What there is, is either in social services records, in the minds of counsellors or in the form of anecdotal evidence taken from professionals on the front line. The fundamental principles of working with child sexual assault are universal. For Black people, the lowering of individual self-esteem is further complicated by the experience of racial hatred, and the social, political and cultural limita-tions imposed upon peoples of African, Caribbean and Asian descent. This is particularly true for the Black child who has suffered sexual assault at the hands of staff in institutions. Anecdotal evidence certainly suggests that such experiences, for a child who is culturally isolated, have sometimes increased the trauma.

Black women have only started using the service to any great degree in the last three years. Work is done with individual women, mothers and their children. We are often given referrals from mental health institutions, social services departments and general practitioners, but our limited resources mean we have been unable to address all requests. Counselling is undertaken only if the woman makes the first appointment herself. We do not counsel women under the influence of drugs or alcohol, or who are undergoing psychiatric or therapeutic treatment.

Over the years I have developed a specific approach to counselling. Its form has been dictated by the resources available and the experiences of women in counselling and psychotherapy. Although it is not definitive it has proved sufficiently useful for the Standing Committee on Sexually

Abused Children to use the basic tenets in its national training programme for professionals working with adult survivors of childhood sexual assault. A number of other agencies have also come to us. Presentations have been made to MIND, the mental health charity, briefings given to lecturers on MSc Social Science programmes, as well as to social services directors across England and to homoeopathy students. This emphasises the far-reaching social implications of the work of the project.

During my work, I have identified a number of reasons why childhood sexual assault takes place. None of them is conclusive; none takes particular note of racial and/or cultural differences. While I cannot discuss these in detail here, I will outline them in order to give context to the approach I have evolved.

The reasons include:

- The 'dysfunctional family' theory, generally subscribed to by social service agencies: this implies collusion on the part of the whole family, and suggests that the abuse is precipitated by the failure of the mother to fulfil her role, either by design or by default.
- The 'Lolita' theory: the concept of a child having a sexual appetite which needs satisfying. It suggests that far from being sexually assaulted by the adult concerned, the adult falls prey to the child's seduction.
- The 'perpetrator profile': a statistical assessment of the social, psychological and physical characteristics of individuals convicted of perpetrating child sexual assault. The information gathered is used to predict the likelihood of another offence being committed.
- The 'feminist' theory that sexual assault is integral to the social mores of patriarchy and the need to maintain the gender power relationships on which it is based.

- The generalised religious belief that perpetrators are evil and that a sin has been committed; in some religious philosophies this implies complicity on the part of the sufferer.

When trying to understand the reasons behind childhood sexual assault, I feel that each concept has a part to play, particularly with respect to the implications for practice. None, however completely answers the question: why does childhood sexual assault take place? Before going any further, it is important to note the influence of Freud[3] in respect to child sexual assault treatment and practice. In 1896, Freud was faced with a Victorian unease about claims of sexual abuse made by many of his female patients against their fathers. As a result, he chose to give public credence to the idea that their allegations were an expression of phantasy, which led to hysteria. The legacy of Freud's capitulation, in terms of treating successive generations of survivors of child sexual assault, has been a commonly held psychiatric view which takes this explanation as its starting point.

Our approach, rather than subscribing to any one theory, attempts to take the most positive features from all of them and relate these to the needs and perceptions of individual women. A complementary aid are the exercises created by Laura Davis and Ellen Bass and published in their book, *The Courage to Heal*. While the book's beginnings are certainly bound in a feminist tradition, it has very clear lines of departure from that tradition.

The curious contradiction is that despite being the ideological force which has brought about the most significant change to date in the field of child sexual abuse, some feminist theory has also served to severely limit the development of work in this area.

Feminism gave voice to the hitherto whispered experience of women who had suffered sexual assault in childhood. Trauma, distress and pain were shared in consciousness-raising groups, challenged in conferences and demonstrations, as well as in letters to television stations and newspapers. Change was realised through the setting up of alternative structures to deal with child sexual assault as part of women's experiences. These included women's centres, rape crisis centres and survivors' support groups. These went on to influence social services departments, the National Health Service, the media, public awareness in general and finally the police and the judiciary. It is to the credit of feminism that in the last ten years we have seen the introduction of the Children Act 1989, child protection teams and a more sensitive police approach to women who have suffered sexual assault.

My work with LRCRP, however, brought me face to face with a feminist theory that has little room for the possibility of women sexual abusers, or for the voice of the boy who has been sexually abused. Nor was there a general comprehension of the fact that childhood sexual assault may not be understood in terms of goodies (women) and (baddies) men. The truth is that a complex network of social, political, economic, spiritual and cultural factors interact to precipitate acts of childhood sexual assault. Somewhere there must be an acknowledgement of the fact that those who have been abused, as well as those who abuse, may be connected to us by blood or association; and that we all have a responsibility to be both vigilant and supportive of everyone involved. These issues have consistently proven to be the Achilles' heel of some feminist theory. There are many debates about each and every one of the theories about the reasons for child sexual assault, and each has its faults and its positive side. Here I have discussed feminist theory because we are a women's organisation working with women and children.

Every woman's experience is different, so our approach provides a framework for dealing with personal distress at a given point in time. Having learned a number of skills during the course of the counselling, the woman may, we hope, return to them at her own choosing. She is taken on a journey of self-investigation, analysis and self-development, which will move at the pace that suits her needs. The process takes six week, after which the woman is advised to take a break for three to six months. It is then suggested that she pursue whatever she considers necessary to ensure her physical, emotional and social well-being.

The programme consists of six hours of counselling. A preliminary meeting is held with the woman to establish whether our method of work will be helpful.

Session one

The woman is encouraged to speak about her experience at her own pace. We try to identify the cause of her anguish: it may be one event, or series of events. Once the source of pain is identified the woman is encouraged to keep a journal and a dream book. The journal may consist of pictures, text or any other means of expression.

Session two

The accumulated material is discussed and the specific area of self-development identified. Personal relationships are looked at, family friends and acquaintances. The journal is used to explore and identify feelings.

Session three

We look at where the woman finds herself now; what her hopes and fears are for the future. What things stop her attaining her goals? The week ahead is devoted to assessing the priorities in her life and setting the wheels of change in motion.

Session four

We look at emotions and their management. Old management styles — for example self-abuse, drugs, alcohol and violence — are looked upon as manifestations of pain. The dream book and journal give the woman an opportunity to monitor her personal coping mechanisms in the week ahead.

Session five

The relationship of significant others — brothers, sisters, lovers, mothers, employers and so on — is explored within the context of the abuse. Affirmations (a method whereby a woman works to change negative feelings into positive ones) are used to explore issues around self-worth and the woman's personal relationships. In the week ahead the woman tests the new self-knowledge she has gained.

Session six

The final session is about disengaging from the counselling relationship. Work is done by the woman to identify where she would like to be a year from now, taking note of her emotions and her ambitions. She draws up a plan to establish how she intends to attain her goals.

Counselling is based on the following assumptions:

- The woman has survived until this point in her life and in so doing has developed a number of skills which may or may not have become outmoded.
- She has come for counselling because in her own assessment there is need for change in her life.
- When in crisis, human beings are vulnerable. The counsellor has an ethical and moral responsibility to have due regard for this fact.
- The counsellor should work to enable the woman to see her strengths.

- The counsellor should respect the differences in the women counselled.
- The time available to the woman is extremely short, six hours in total. The counsellor should selectively use professional experience and information to highlight commonalities (with the experiences of other women survivors) and validate the individual's experience. (This should be done without self-disclosure, as this can result in the time being used for the counsellor's benefit.)
- The counsellor's role is to listen, to hear, to reflect and to generate thought and questions in the women using the service.
- Trauma often induces a pattern of frozen negativity. The counsellor should take nothing for granted about the way individual's lives are lived.
- The counsellor should respect the woman's perspective about her experience.

At the end of 1992 Lambeth Women and Children's Health Project ran a training course for women interested in counselling women who have suffered sexual assault in childhood. The project now has eight trainee counsellors from a wide variety of cultural and social backgrounds. They were trained by myself and Kate Gledhill, using a programme we designed, to introduce and make more widely available the approach that has just been outlined. There are plans to update a small pamphlet published by the project entitled *You and Your Child: For Mothers of Children who have been Sexually Abused* by Patricia Agana, Kate Gledhill, Carole Ann Hooper and Jackie Pearce. The aim is to bring it into line with current legislation such as the Children Act 1989.

There is still an absence of research on the incidence and prevalence of sexual assault in childhood in minority communities. So what is current practice based upon? We may well ask! This anomaly remains a challenge to the project, and to all those interested in developing the work. In the meantime, racial negatives are a complicating factor in the management of childhood sexual assault. The work of the Lambeth Women and Children's Health Project is a small step towards the provision of a service which addresses the cultural needs of all our communities.

Notes

1. 'Nobody', by Brenda Hayde-Agard, in *Times Like These*, Obatala Press, 1988. Copies may be purchased from the Lambeth Women and Children's Health Project.
2. OWAAD (Organisation of Women of African and Asian Descent) is addressed in *Heart of the Race* by Bryan, Dadzie and Scafe (Virago, 1985).
3. J. Masson (1992) *The Assault on Truth, Freud and Child Sexual Abuse*, Fontana 1992, London.

A Needle in a Haystack:
Finding Support as a Survivor of
Domestic Violence

Antoinette Clark

> 'Today, I have come out of my husband's jail and entered the
> jail of the law. But I have found a new life, in the legal jail.
> It's in this cage that I found a kind of freedom.'
>
> (*Women Against Fundamentalism*, 1992–3)

This quote is from a statement made by Kiranjit Ahluwalia
during her life imprisonment for setting fire to her violent
husband. She was freed after Southall Black Sisters and
other women's groups mounted a campaign to illustrate
the way the legal system condemns women to remain in
violent relationships. Kiranjit was released at the Old
Bailey on September 25, 1993 after she pleaded manslaughter on grounds of diminished responsibility. (*Women
Against Fundamentalism*, 1992–3)

This chapter focuses on the problems Black women have
in finding support from both legal and counselling services.
I shall explore these services and what access Black women
have to them. I have concentrated on self help. Good health
is about taking charge. This chapter charts the methods
given to us as women to use to escape domestic violence.

The Home Office statistics for homicide show that 25
per cent of all murders are domestic. Seventy women a year
are killed by their male partners while only 12 men a year

are killed by the women they have been abusing. Forty per cent of men who kill get their conviction reduced to manslaughter, usually on the ground of provocation. Provocation means that a woman has provoked her husband or boyfriend to kill her by 'nagging', 'refusing to have sex' and 'behaving badly'. (*Rights of Women*: 1992)

This has been an uneasy piece to write. For starters, I am having to review my own personal experiences of domestic violence and having to re-live the abuse I experienced at the hands of my ex-partner. I am also reminded of the lack of legal information available to me during that time.

Secondly, there is generally a lack of research which focuses on Black women's situation. Feminism has centralised its campaign on the resistance of male violence. Male violence is seen as the power of men to control women. As a Black feminist, I found this analysis problematic as it does not include all the types of violence I have experienced, including that of racist attacks in which both white men and women have participated (Mama: 1989). Feminist theory has reflected mainly white, middle class women's thinking, while Black radical politics reflect Black male thoughts. Black women are forced to choose whether to follow our race or our gender politics separately. There will be some who find my reflections too simplistic or not politically engaging on this point.

Thirdly, there is a problem of my own self esteem. Writing is a vulnerable act. There is a lot of intellectual policing which occurs within the feminist community. Therefore, I preface this piece by saying it is one advice worker's experience of working with women. As an advice worker I am supposed to impart to 'clients' knowledge of the laws, the policies of social services departments, the safety of different forms of counselling and therapy and the ability of the police and courts to act effectively and fairly. Any advice I give must be impartial and lawful. How is this possible in a legal system which ignores women's rights?

Women who have tried to leave a violent partner will know how difficult this really can be. The abuse a woman sustains is not only physical and sexual, but also involves continual emotional and psychological undermining, which the abuser uses to remain in charge. The question, for those who don't understand the nature of abuse is, 'Why don't the women just leave?' In order for a woman to 'leave' her abuser, she must escape. In Kiranjit's case, the only escape possible was to kill her violent husband. Abusers tell women that they will never get away; that their husband/partner will find them wherever they go. Many abusers are powerful men with access to information and resources to track women down. Even when men are not powerful in their everyday lives, a lack of resources and laws and religion which makes it a duty to stay with a violent man mean that women are trapped by circumstance.

I am not advocating that women kill their partners as a means of escape. I do want to pursue questions of 'What solutions are left when you fear for your life and the lives of your children?' 'What do you do when all legal and counselling solutions have failed?' Many women in violent situations feel they have few choices. They try the ways offered to them. They get injunctions, go into therapy, call the police. They go to refuges and still they feel they are under threat. Women are forced to maintain arrangements for abusers to see children. The courts, in insisting that women stick to these arrangements, separate children's and women's interests. The reasoning seems to be that just because a woman has been beaten, stabbed or verbally assaulted does not mean that a father can be denied access to his child. Children's welfare is defined as needing fathers at all costs, including women's lives.

I define domestic violence as the physical, emotional and sexual abuse of a person in what is meant to be a trusted, safe and intimate relationship. The abuse is defined by the person who is experiencing the abuse and not by the abuser's perception of his/her actions. The legal definition speaks in terms of 'victims', 'men and women', 'marriage' and 'evidence'. It is perceived that a woman must be living with her husband. Violence occurs to women whether they are living with their abusers or not. It also occurs between women in lesbian relationships. It can occur even when the man has not left marks which the courts can interpret as evidence. 'Domestic' denotes something private and out of the public eye. A woman is told by her abuser not to tell anyone of her abuse because she will never be believed. In my view, the legal system supports the abuser's position.

The type of support a woman can expect will fit broadly into four categories:

1. The law which is not only the laws themselves, but the interpretation of law and those involved in the processes of law including the police, courts, and lawyers.
2. Counselling and advice-giving agencies. These include Citizens' Advice Bureaux, Rape Crisis Centres and marriage guidance. There are also private counsellors, therapists and women's centres.
3. The local authority provides a whole range of services, from housing to social services, which includes daycare. The local authority also has legal powers relating to investigating the protection of children from abuse.
4. The Benefits Agency, which gives women access to financial assistance.

A woman's experience of domestic violence is a mixture of alarm and of not being taken seriously. The police describe a woman being abused in her own home as a 'domestic'. What this means to me is that it is okay for an abuser to assault their partner at home because such affairs are a private matter. The police have begun to set up units to help women who are experiencing violence, but there is still a gap between the police intentions and the service that women receive from the police. As a Black woman, it is very difficult for me to decide what involvement the police should have in any affair. The worry of further violence from the police makes Black women unsure about police involvement.

I have provided a brief outline of legal rights for women who want to escape domestic violence. The law is constructed to keep women and children within the control of men. As Black women we are kept ignorant of our legal rights. While some of us know how to 'play' the system, many do not understand what the system is and how it operates. As a child, I grew up with the notion that the worst thing that could happen to a Black woman and her children was to have white social workers poking their noses around in their lives. The law, in the experience of Black people, represents trouble or being in trouble; it is not regarded as something to be 'used' in our defence. It was not until this century that Black women were able to use the law in their own interests. Until then white men physically owned us and we had no status in law (Williams, 1993).

Now that we have gained our rights, some of us may feel we can use the law as a method of gaining justice. The law is not about being just or fair. The law is a set of rules society invents to maintain the particular way the society wishes to be organised at any time. Laws are the written rules. Lawyers present their view of the rules in relationship to their client's situation. Courts decide whose view is more reasonable.

Black women's participation in the legal profession is invisible. We are inhibited from being lawyers because of the racism and sexism of the legal profession. When we use white solicitors and barristers, their interaction with us can often be quite negative. They may misrepresent us, not obey our wishes or deny us information. They may be slow with processes relating to our case. Our access can also be barred because of language, partly because many of us speak English as a second language. Where does this book fit into that? But also the law is not conducted in everyday speech. At Rights of Women, a lot of my time was spent explaining what things meant, whether it was solicitors' letters, orders from the court, or affidavits. Because we do not understand what is being said about us, it makes it difficult for us to defend our interests.

Giving legal advice is controversial. I am not sure, for instance, by the time this is published how much of it will be applicable. What use is this guide, if what I am constantly pointing out is that there is no justice in the system. I was involved in a volunteer feminist project which supported women who suffered violence. It was a policy not to inform Black women about the range of legal remedies they could use. It was felt that the law was racist and that Black women would only encounter more racist abuse by using the legal process. I was angry. White feminists, with the best intentions, take this stand on the grounds of protecting us. What they don't realise is that their attitude is racist. It is up to us to decide whether or not we wish to use the courts to protect us.

In the case of Kiranjit Ahluwalia, a campaign was started to change the law to release her from prison. Kiranjit tried to defend herself by pouring petrol on her husband's feet and legs while he was lying down and setting light to it with a match. Her defence for doing this was that she had just wanted to injure him to stop him coming after her. Several days later, he died from his wounds. A campaign spurred by Kiranjit's case was mounted on behalf of women who killed their abusive partners. It sought to change the law so that women who killed their husbands in self defence were not tried for murder. Pressure was placed on both the government and judiciary to have an understanding of what the lives of women who live in violent domestic situations is really like.

The reality is that there are not enough services for women who experience violence. We need a whole range of services from police protection, to laws which remove the abuser (instead of us) from the home, as well as support, counselling, emergency childcare, education, training and financial support so that we can start new and independent lives, act in any domestic circumstance, including one involving a lesbian relationship. I have tried to outline the politics of our lives to provide a framework for understanding why anything we receive in the way of services will be because we have fought for them: fought not only our abusers, but also the very people who keep telling us they are trying to help.

HOW TO ESCAPE

Get help and keep safe

Leaving a violent situation is extremely difficult. Don't let anyone tell you it isn't. The first thing that must be uppermost in your mind is: how do I get out? The following guide is to help you. Not everything you need to know is here, but it does give an idea of the types of thing you will have to do to escape.

Step one

Be calculating. Plan your escape, whether this means having your partner removed from the home, or you going. If you are leaving your home, this might take several attempts. Each time you try and go back you will probably feel like a failure. If the courts, social workers and police are already involved, a tremendous amount of guilt and pressure will be placed on you about wasting their time. At this point you will probably be considering many aspects of your future, such as housing, children, finances and survival in general.

Step two: 'to stay' or 'to go'

Each way carries its own brand of trauma. The system, a real sixties word, is only interested in you to the extent that you are a problem. In realistic terms, you can expect the worst accommodation, both temporary and permanent. You may also find that many professionals are not always supportive. Domestic violence is an industry in which careers are made and where there are many 'experts'. Do not rely on their help fully, and any time someone tells you something which does not feel right, check it out. Your fate is in your own hands. Like everyone else, professionals are stretched because of a lack of resources and imagination. The last thing you want is to be landed with someone whose own personal crisis seems to be greater than yours. Whichever way you decide, there are basic things you must remember:

1. Nobody deserves to be treated as you have been or are being treated. If you are reading this chapter to gain help/strength/ideas about how to get out of a violent situation, tell yourself: don't just read about it, take a step towards doing it.

2. It is OK to feel a lot of mixed emotions about your partner. There will be feelings of great love and great anger. You might even feel that you did 'something' to cause your partner to be so abusive towards you. You will rack your brain for some clue. You might even want to return so that you can reason with your partner and make it better. You

are not the problem. Your partner is. You are not safe staying together any longer.

3. Talk to anybody who will listen. Your abuser wants you to keep it a secret. This is particularly relevant in Black communities, where we feel that we should keep our problems to ourselves for fear of what white folks will think about us. The more people you tell, the more you will discover how common your situation really is. As Black women we exist in isolation, apart from our families, with white neighbours who may either abuse us or ignore us. But we must break our silence. We must create avenues so that we can talk and discuss. One of my most memorable experiences is of a client who was a mum at a school. She spoke to me because she and a group of other mums wanted to learn how to support another woman who was being abused. Talk to everyone – you never know where you will gain support.

4. Protect your children and do not endure the situation any longer for their sake. If you feel unsafe, they will feel unsafe, too. This is contrary to legal opinion, which feels that fathers should be given contact/access to their children, no matter what they have done to the mother. If you leave and take your children, you must protect yourself from the authorities. You can do this by taking legal advice immediately or by informing your solicitor before you leave with the children. The solicitor will inform your partner that the children are safe and can start to take immediate proceedings against him. This safeguards you against allegations of abduction. If you decide to leave your children you must establish that they will be safe while they are not in your care. Your children will have no resources to keep themselves safe when you are not there.

There are two main pieces of legislation concerning children which you may want to read and discuss further with a legal adviser:

The Children Act 1989 (the legal advice service Rights of Women has a good simple leaflet discussing the Act): this describes parents' responsibilities and how the law mediates between parents when the relationship has broken down. The Act strengthens fathers' responsibilities. I would say rights, but the Act is not specifically about parents' rights, but about what is in the best interests of the child. Unmarried fathers, in certain instances, have just as many rights as married fathers. This change will affect Black women's lives dramatically since many of us do not choose to marry the fathers of our children. The Act makes no direct reference to women experiencing domestic violence. Some men have used the Act and its pro-father stance to gain access to women.

The Child Support Act 1991: this states that both parents have a legal responsibility to support their children. If you are on benefit, you will be required to pursue the father for maintenance. If you are trying to hide or want to have very little contact with your partner because of violence, this Act will make it very difficult. There is, however, an important exception made by the Act. If contact with the father will cause you to suffer harm or undue distress as set out under Section 6(2), then you will not be required to find him. The Child Support Agency will not disclose your whereabouts to the other parent without your permission. Do not count on this. It is important to have evidence of the abuse you have suffered to convince these agencies of the urgency of your situation.

5. Always go for medical treatment any time violence of any description occurs to you or your children. Not only will this serve as a record, but you must ensure that your health and well-being is as good as it can be. Internal bruis-

ing and fractures are common and must receive medical attention. The doctor has to keep affairs related to your health confidential, but does not have to keep the details of your child/children confidential. He or she will be required to tell the local authority of any abuse that is discovered. This may seem harsh, but it is better to be aware of the situation concerning your children than to have the social services discover it through other sources such as schools and teachers. Black family life is always being scrutinised: professionals expect us to abuse our children, especially physically. They feel it is a part of our 'culture' to be harsh and brutal disciplinarians.

6. Get a solicitor or seek legal advice from a law centre, even if you are not going to follow that advice at the time. If you are on income support you are entitled to legal aid. If you are working, ask the solicitor first what the costs will be so that you can see whether you can afford their fees. You might be entitled to some legal aid, but that will have to be worked out with the solicitor. Do not automatically use the solicitor on your local high street. Make sure you get one who is recommended by either a friend or an agency, and who is experienced in family law, domestic violence and Black women's issues. Visit a few and then make your decision. This person will be very important in your life, so choose someone you feel comfortable with. Before you visit the solicitor, write your story down from the start of the relationship, with details of all incidents of abuse, including all injuries you have suffered. Include any kind of harassment including phone calls, notes and threatening behaviour. Also include all the times you have sought medical attention, rung the police or visited the social services. If you haven't done this up until now, keep a diary. If you are still living with the abuser make sure your diary is locked away in a place he or she can't find. In the diary include emergency numbers of organisations like the National Federation of Women's Aid, Rights of

Women, Rape Crisis, Lesbian and Gay Switchboard, the Samaritans and the nearest Citizens' Advice Bureau or other advice centre. Refer to the list at the end of this book for numbers of organisations that will give you free emergency support.

7. You are entitled to claim income support from the moment your partner leaves you or you leave the home. Be prepared to explain your situation. In certain circumstances even if you have 'no recourse to public funds' you can claim them at a reduced rate. You must take further advice, as the DSS will inform the Home Office. This has been extremely difficult for Black women who were brought to this country by husbands who have violently abused them. If you have lived here under a year, are no longer living with your husband, and are forced to claim benefits because you cannot work, you can be deported. Black women who have this status stamped in their passport can also be deported if seeking rehousing and/or are claiming housing benefit in order to stay in a bed and breakfast. If you are such a woman, please seek advice before you claim anything.

Step three: 'to go'
Pack these things before you go (sometimes it is difficult to get them after you leave).

1. Birth certificates, both yours and the children's. The children's birth certificates are very important. Believe it or not, you might have to prove the children are yours. Some housing authorities seem to believe that Black women are 'borrowing' children to get housing.

2. Marriage certificate, if there is one.

3. Favourite photographs.

4. Inventory of all the items of furniture and accessories in your house and who purchased them. Give this to your solicitor. You will want to negotiate about what items you want to take. Don't do yourself out of anything just because

the property is still in the house. Remember, you have to start again, and rebuilding a home is a very expensive business. Carry out these negotiations quickly so that your partner does not have time to damage things. Even if you are in a bed and breakfast the DSS can pay to have your things removed and put into storage until you are rehoused. The local authority, however, will not necessarily rehouse you unless you have children with you. Although grants are available they are quite hard to get and can take a long time. Tactically, it is a good idea to apply for both a crisis/budgeting loan and a community care grant at the same time because you can get a crisis loan immediately whilst a community care grant may take months. In the meantime you will be required to pay the loan back. If you have been on income support for less that 26 weeks you will not be able to get a budgeting loan. Community care grants and crisis loans *do not* require you to be on income support, although the DSS are likely to tell you otherwise. Get further advice. Do not be put off if you are refused; always ask for a review. After two requests, if you are still not happy with the decision, the DSS has to pass your case to a social fund inspector who really is independent of the DSS.

5. All items relating to financial matters – saving books, chequebooks, cheque/cash cards, bank statements, benefit books and so on.

6. All items relating to housing matters – mortgage information, rent books, tenancy agreements and so on.

7. Passports.

8. All documents from the Home Office. These are important if you are going to claim benefits in your own right, especially if you have come to the country in the past five years.

9. Inform the gas, electric, and telephone companies as soon as you go, so that if you return you cannot be held liable for services used during your absence. Tell British

Telecom not to send an itemised bill, and why. This is so that your abuser cannot find out where you are from the numbers of the people you have been ringing.

10. Address book – so that your abuser can't track you down.

11. Jewellery.

12. The children's favourite toys and clothing.

13. Sentimental treasures. Partners will often destroy these after you have gone.

14. Copies of all solicitors' letters, including any court orders you have been granted such as injunctions and orders related to the care of your children.

15. Prescribed medicines.

Step four: 'to stay'

It is possible to get protection from the courts to stay in your house. Under the Domestic Violence and Matrimonial Proceedings Act 1976 any woman, married or unmarried, may obtain an injunction in the county court against her male partner. An injunction can also be sought (although these are extremely rare and difficult to get) against other members of the family including older male children, parents and in-laws. An injunction is a court order that requires the man not to harass, threaten or molest you. Usually, injunctions will exclude a partner either from part of the home where you reside, or from the entire home, or it will order the partner to keep several miles away from the home. You may get an injunction even if the home is solely in the man's name. A married woman may apply to the magistrates' court. An injunction, in order to be effective, should include the power of arrest, as the police are slow to act on injunctions that do not include this. An exclusion order with powers of arrest is hard to get, but it is possible if your solicitor perseveres. Courts like there to have been some actual physical harm or what they consider a real threat to a woman's life. An injunction can be obtained within two days, but you can get an emergency injunction within 24 hours. You will need a solicitor to do this.

During the first few days or weeks it is important to find several people who are willing to stay with you until you feel your ex-partner will not visit you again. You can also ask for your telephone number to be changed, and to be ex-directory. Alternatively, an operator can screen your calls. If the violence does not cease, it might be important for you to rethink your decision to stay. While none of us want to lose our homes, and it is difficult to find another, it is more important to be safe.

If you have a mortgage the DSS can pay the interest on the whole loan whether the house is in joint names or in the man's name only, in order to keep you there. Take further legal advice on this.

WHERE YOU CAN GO TO FIND SUPPORT FOR ESCAPING

The police

The police have never been our best friends. But who else can we turn to when we need support? Some police stations now have domestic violence suites with trained officers. I have interviewed and met policemen and women in these suites. On the whole, they do provide a service and they are trying to understand the problems women face. It is best to locate one of these units, if your local police station doesn't have one.

With the police, you have the right to a quick and sensitive response and also the right to ask to talk to a woman police officer; for your partner to be interviewed separately from you; for additional local sources of help and support, including negotiation with local authorities; for transportation to a women's refuge or any other place you feel safe; and for help to re-enter your home so that you can remove your belongings.

The caring professionals

These include counsellors, doctors, therapists, helplines and advice agencies. I belong to this category of professionals, with which must come a general health warning. There will be many who will strongly disagree with my position. Counselling and therapy can be an empowering experience but, at certain points in life, it can be a debilitating one too, depending on the counsellor and methods used. Any counsellor you choose should have a good understanding both of women's issues and of Black women's experience of oppression. This applies to both Black and white counsellors. The aim of counselling at this time should be to allow you to cope and make decisions about today.

We have a long way to go before we get services which reflect our needs. My heartfelt advice is to be what white folks and our ex-partners always fear from Black women – that loud, screaming and demanding nightmare they dread.

References

1. K. Ahluwalia, 'Kiranjit Ahluwalia Wins Freedom,' *Women Against Fundamentalism*, Volume 4, Winter, 1992–93, p. 1.
2. J. Radford, 'Self-Preservation, Proposal for a New Defence to the Charge of Murder,' *Rights of Women*, Summer Bulletin, 1992, p. 6.
3. A. Mama, *The Hidden Struggle: Statutory and Voluntary Responses to Violence Against Black Women*, London, Runnymede Trust, 1989.
4. P. Williams, *The Alchemy of Race and Rights*, Virago Press, 1993.

Taking the Home Out of Homophobia: Black Lesbian Health

Jewelle L. Gomez and Barbara Smith

Without the licence to give breath to all our dimensions, it is impossible for black women to achieve true health. For black lesbians, anti-gay sentiments compound the racism and sexism that circumscribe all black female lives. In the following piece, two black lesbian writers discuss the debilitating toll homophobia takes on black gays. Furthermore, they challenge blacks to address and relinquish the oppressive religious traditions that have historically made homosexuality taboo in our community.

Barbara: One of the things we've been asked to talk about is how homophobia affects Black women's mental health. I think that in addition to affecting lesbians' emotional health, homophobia also affects the mental health of heterosexual people. In other words, being homophobic is not a healthy state for people to be in.

Jewelle: I'd like to hear more about that.

Barbara: Well, it's just like being a racist. I don't think that most Blacks or other people of colour would vouch for the mental health of somebody who is a rabid and snarling racist. Because that's like dismissing a part of the human family. Particularly within the African-American community, when we are so embattled, it's just baloney to dismiss or say that a certain segment is expendable because of their sexual orientation. Anyone who would do that hasn't grown up, they're just not mature.

Jewelle: I think it's even more dangerous for people of colour to embrace homophobia than it is for whites to embrace racism, simply because we're embattled psychologically and economically as an ethnic group. We leave ourselves in a very weakened position if we allow the system to pit us against each other. I also think it renders Black people politically smug. That's the thing about homophobia, racism, anti-Semitism, any of the 'isms' – once you embrace those you tend to become smug.

And once you take a position of smugness you lose your fighting edge. I think African-Americans who've taken the position of 'we are the major victim' in this society and nobody else has suffered like we've suffered, lose their edge. They don't have the perspective that will allow us to fight through all the issues.

Barbara: Right. From the time we get here, we are steeped in the knowledge that we are the victims of a really bigoted and racist society. But we also have to acknowledge that there are ways that we can be oppressive to other groups whose identities we don't share. So I think that one of the challenges we face in trying to raise the issue of lesbian and gay identity within the Black community is to try to get our people to understand that they can indeed oppress someone after having spent a life of being oppressed. That's a very hard transition to make, but it's one we have to make if we want our whole community to be liberated.

Jewelle: At this point it seems almost impossible because the issue of sexism has become such a major stumbling block for the Black community. I think we saw the beginning of it in the 1970s with Ntozake Shange's play, *For Colored Girls Who Have Considered Suicide/When the Rainbow Is Enuf*. The play really prompted Black women to embrace the idea of independent thinking; to begin looking to

186

each other for sustenance and to start appreciating and celebrating each other in ways that we've always done naturally. I think that the Black male community was so horrified to discover that they were not at the centre of Black women's thoughts that they could only perceive the play as a negative attack upon them. I think that for the first time, that play made the Black community look at its sexism. And many people rejected Ntozake Shange and things having to do with feminism in a very cruel way. So years later, when we got the Central Park incident with the white woman being beaten and raped by a group of young Black males, all people could talk about was the role racism played in the attack.

Barbara: I happened to be at a writers' retreat in April 1989 when that incident occurred. It was a radicalised retreat run by a group of old lefties, so everybody there had to have a certain level of political consciousness. There was one woman there who had been involved in progressive politics for decades and she and I were discussing the Central Park rape. Her sole concern was whether these young Black and Latino men were going to get a fair trial. I couldn't believe what I was hearing. And I thought, this is why a Black feminist analysis is so important. It's important because my concern was that there was a woman lying up in the hospital almost dead. A woman who if she ever recovers physically, is likely to be profoundly psychologically damaged for the rest of her life. Black feminism is important because we can look at these issues from a holistic and principled perspective as opposed to a reductive one.

There was an article in the *Village Voice* in which some Black women were asked what they thought about the Central Park rape and most of them came down very hard on sexual violence and sexism in the Black community. They indeed cited sexism as a cause of the rape. This incident is not a mysterious fluke. It is part and parcel of what African-American women face on the streets and in their homes every day. There was a Black woman standing in a supermarket line right here in New York City and they were talking about the rape. There was a Black man behind her and he was apparently wondering why they had to beat the white woman, why they had to do her like that. And then he said, 'Why didn't they just rape her?' As if that would have been OK. So you see, we have a lot to contend with.

Jewelle: I think that the sexism continues to go un-acknowledged and even praised as part of the Black community's survival technique. The subsequent acceptance of homophobia that falls naturally with that kind of thinking will be the thing that cripples the Black community. During the civil rights movement, it was a single focus on desegregation that gave us an impetus to move and hold on to our vision. But it is that same single focus that has left us with these half-assed solutions to our problems today. I mean a movement towards the middle class is not a solution to the problems in the Black community. And I think it's just pathetic that the narrowness of vision in the African-American community has left us with that. Therefore, it's not surprising that homophobia is part of the fallout. Nor should people be surprised about the anti-Semitism in the Black community. It's just one more of the 'isms' that xenophobic oppressed groups justify themselves in taking on simply because they are oppressed groups.

Barbara: Right.

Jewelle: It's been said that people to whom evil has been done, will do evil in return.

Barbara: Who said that?

Jewelle: W. H. Auden. So I don't think we should be surprised about homophobia. It sneaks up in a very subtle and destructive way, even though homosexuality has always been an intrinsic part of the Black community.

Barbara: Absolutely.

Jewelle: When I was growing up, everyone always knew who was gay. When the guys came to my father's bar, I knew which ones were gay, it was clear as day. For instance, there was Miss Kay who was a big queen and Maurice. These were people that everybody knew. They came and went in my father's bar just like everybody else. This was a so-called lower-class community – the working poor in Boston. It was a community in which people did not talk about who was gay, but I knew who the lesbians were. It was always unspoken and I think that there's something about leaving it unspoken that leaves us unprepared.

Barbara: That's the breakpoint for this part of the twentieth century as far as I'm concerned. There've been lesbian and gay men, Black ones, as long as there've been African people. So that's not even a question. You know how they say that the human race was supposed to have been started by a Black woman? Well, since she had so many children, some of them were undoubtedly queer. [*Laughter.*] Writer Ann Allen Shockley has a wonderful line about that which I use often. 'Play it, but don't say it.' That's the sentiment that encapsulates the general stance of the Black community on sexual identity and orientation. If you're a lesbian, you can have as many women as you want. If you're a gay man, you can have all the men you want. But just don't say anything about it or make it political. The difference today is that the lesbian and gay movement prides itself on being out, verbalising one's identity and organising around our oppression. With the advent of this movement, the African-American community has really been confronted with some stuff that they've never had to deal with before.

I grew up in Cleveland in a community very similar to the one you described. Today the issue is not whether gay people have been here since for ever. It's that we are telling our community that it has to deal with us differently than before. That's what contemporary Black gay and lesbian activists are doing.

Jewelle: I was thinking, as you were saying that, that if one embraces the principles of liberation, gay liberation and feminism, then you have to assault the sexual stereotype that young Black girls have been forced to live out in the African-American community. The stereotype that mandates that you develop into the well-groomed girl who pursues a profession and a husband.

Barbara: High achiever.

Jewelle: Or the snappy baby machine. You tend to go one way or the other. You're either fast or you're well groomed. I think that for so many young Black women, the idea of finding their place in society has been defined by having a man or a baby. So if you begin to espouse a proud lesbian growth, you find yourself going against the grain. That makes embracing your lesbianism doubly frightening, because you then have to discard the mythology that's been developed around what it means to be a young Black woman.

Barbara: And that you gotta have a man. The urgency of which probably can't even be conveyed on the printed page. [*Laughter.*] I was just going to talk about when I was younger and meeting people who would want to know about me. Not so much about my sexual orientation, because they weren't even dealing with the fact that somebody could be a lesbian. But I always noticed they were more surprised to find out I didn't have children than that I wasn't married. Marriage was not the operative thing. It was like, 'Why don't you have any children?' That really made them curious.

Jewelle: Right. They had no understanding at all that you could reach a certain age and not have any children.

Barbara: And not having children doesn't mean we're selfish. It means we're self-referenced. Many Black lesbians and gay men have children. Those of us who don't may not have had the opportunity. Or we may have made the conscious choice not to have children.

One of the things about being a Black lesbian is that we're very conscious. At least those of us who are politicised about what we will and will not have in our lives. Coming out is such a conscious choice that the process manifests itself in other areas of our lives.

Jewelle: Yes, it's healthy. Having grown up with a lot of Black women who had children at an early age, I've noticed a contradictory element in that that's the way many of them come into their own. I have younger cousins who have two, three, four children and are not married and will probably never be married. It seems that the moment they have the baby is when they come into their own and their identity after that becomes the 'long-suffering Black mother'. I think it recreates a cycle of victimisation because a lot of these young women carry the burden of being on a road that wasn't really a conscious choice. On the other hand, when I look at Black lesbian mothers, I see that yes, many of them are struggling with their children. But there is also a sense of real choice because they've made a conscious decision to be out and have children. They are not long-suffering victims. They are not women who have been abandoned by their men. They are lesbian mothers who have made a place in the world that is not a victim's place. Now that doesn't necessarily mean that things are any easier or simpler for them. But there is a psychological difference because most Black lesbian mothers have made a choice and have a community they can look to for support.

Barbara: In talking about choice, another thing we've been asked to address is why do people become lesbians, or why did we become lesbians, or why do we think there is such a thing as lesbianism?

Jewelle: It was all those vegetables. Eating too much spinach. [*Laughter.*]

Barbara: Well, I was a notorious non-vegetable eater all my life. Maybe it was the candy bars in my case. Seriously, I don't know why people are lesbians. All I want to say is that I think the reason women become lesbians is because they are deeply attracted – sexually – to other women. To me, that's the bottom line. There was a notion during the early women's movement, in which I was involved, that you could choose to be a lesbian. But I think the important point is whether you choose to be out, or to act on your lesbian feelings. Those of us who were coming out before there was a women's or lesbian and gay movement, understand this a little bit better. I teach students who are in their early twenties and they really perceive their coming out as say, a political choice because they are doing it in such a supportive context. Those of us who were coming out just before Stonewall knew that we had feelings, passion and lust for other women.[1] We didn't necessarily have a place for our feelings that felt safe. But we knew intuitively – not because we read it in a book somewhere – that gay was good. Today people have women's studies courses, out lesbian teachers, all kinds of stuff that we didn't have. So they can indeed perceive their coming out as following in the footsteps of a role model.

Jewelle: I grew up in a bar community and I knew I was a lesbian when I was quite young. But the only available role models weren't anything like who I thought I was going to be when I grew up. I knew I wasn't going to be sitting up in a bar all day, or hustling on the streets. So what was I going to be? There were no other role models.

Barbara: That was the complete terror. Talking about how being a lesbian and homophobia affect one's mental health – I lived my adolescence and young adulthood in terror. I knew I was a lesbian, too. But likewise, I saw no way to act on it and stay on the path. This was a path that I had not necessarily chosen for myself, but that my family had worked very hard to give me the option of choosing. I'd think, How the hell can I excel in school, go to college, graduate school – and then become low life by sleeping with women? I mean it just didn't jibe. Some people think that when I came out during the women's movement it was an easy thing. But I'd just like to say right here for the record, that from puberty on, I had screaming nightmares because I was having dreams of being sexual with women. I would wake up and my grandmother would be standing looking over me and I thought she knew what I was dreaming. She knew that I was disturbed about something, even though I never revealed to her what it was. So, I was really terrified.

I think that conscious lesbianism lived in the context of community is a positive thing. It can be a really affirming choice for women. The connection to sexism is deep, though. Homophobia is a logical extension of sexual oppression because sexual oppression is about roles – one gender does this, the other does that. One's on top, the other is on the bottom.

Jewelle: I think the interconnection of racism and sexism has been so profound that we don't even know how the homophobia is going to be difficult for us as Black women. I've just recently begun to separate them out. I didn't really come out through the women's movement. For me, my sexuality didn't have a political context until later. I always had a sexual identity that I tried to sift out, but I was most concerned about how I was going to fit it in with being a Black Catholic which was very difficult. Once I realised that one of them had to go – sexuality or Catholicism – it took me about five or ten minutes to drop Catholicism. [*Laughter.*] Then I focused on racism, to the exclusion of homophobia and everything else. That left me unprepared. I had a woman lover very early. Then I slept with men until my mid-twenties. They were kind of like the entertainment until I found another girlfriend and got my bearings. I didn't have the political context to deal with what it meant to want to sleep with both men and women. I skipped past the feminism until much later. So homophobia came as a total shock to me because I had never experienced it. Nobody seemed to be homophobic in my community, because no one ever talked about it. I hadn't experienced it because I wasn't out. I didn't know that I wasn't out. But I wasn't.

Barbara: Because you weren't out, you weren't really experiencing homophobia consciously.

Jewelle: Right. I thought it was an aberration. I didn't quite understand what it meant. It reminded me of the first time I heard about child abuse. That happened when I was a teenager and I thought child abuse could only have happened once or twice in the history of the world because it was so appalling to me and beyond my comprehension. And of course as I read more and realised it was –

Barbara: Pandemic.

Jewelle: Yes. I had to withdraw for a little bit to figure it out. It seemed as if someone had just stabbed me in my heart. I think I felt the same way when I understood there was such a thing as homophobia. A couple of years ago, I had an eye-opening experience while looking for an apartment in Jersey City. Now, I had experienced racism in Manhattan. In fact, someone had told me that when I called for an apartment not to reveal my last name because Manhattan landlords would think I was Puerto Rican.

Barbara: This is America.

Jewelle: So I'd just say that my name was Jewelle and show up at the apartment. This was in the early 1970s and it seemed that back then, being Black was a little bit more acceptable than being Puerto Rican, so they would rent to me. And also because I worked for television at that time, the landlords somehow took that to mean that I was OK, that I was better than just the average 'Joe Blackperson' off the streets.

But looking for an apartment in Jersey City with my then lover, who was Black, was very different. Frequently, we'd be dealing with people who had two-family homes and were looking to rent one of the units. I remember we called this one place, and I was in stark terror. In my mind, I was thinking about a white couple looking at us and seeing two Black people that they were going to potentially bring into their home. It terrified me because I could see them insulting us or even possibly slamming the door in our face. And then just as we were about to get out of the car, it occurred to me that this white couple would also look at us and see two lesbians.[*Laughter.*] I was literally shaking. I had been so focused on them seeing two Black women that it hadn't occurred to me that they would also see two lesbians. They'd see the quintessential butch–femme couple, both of us going into our forties.

Barbara: Yes. Well beyond the college room–mate stage.

Jewelle: It terrified me. But as it turns out, they would have rented to us if we had decided to take the place, which we didn't. But the anxiety I suffered during those minutes before we rang the doorbell was devastating and definitely scarred me internally.

Barbara: Of course. It's deep. This is one of the permutations of how homophobia and heterosexism overshadow our lives. One of the things that I'm very happy about now is that I live in Albany, New York. And they did allow me to buy a house there. I don't know how many Chase Manhattans I would have had to rob down here in New York City in order to get enough money to buy a house. [*Laughter.*] My house is in the heart of Albany's Black community. And one of the really nice things about it is that I know that nobody can put me out of my house because of what I have on my walls, who I bring in there, or whatever. That's very refreshing. Of course, it's the first time I've ever felt that way. What I'd always done before, because of homophobia and racism, was to be pretty low-key wherever I lived. I just felt that around my house, I had to try to be very cautious, even though I'm known to be a very out lesbian, both politically and in print. I didn't want anybody following me into my house who thought that bulldaggers shouldn't be allowed to live.

Jewelle: I know. When the plumber is coming to my Brooklyn apartment to fix something, all of my lesbian things get put away.

Barbara: Because he knows where you live and may even have a key to the apartment.

Jewelle: Yes. I have no desire to wake up and discover the plumber and his helper standing over me.

Barbara: That's right. That's real. This gets into an area that is very important for all people, especially Black people in this country, to understand. And that is that we pay a heavy toll for being who we are and living with integrity. Being out means you are doing what your grandmother told you to do, which is not to lie. Black lesbians and gays who are out are not lying. But we pay high prices for our integrity. People really need to understand that there is entrenched violence against lesbians and gay men that is much like and parallel to the racial violence that has characterised Black people's lives since we've been in this country. When we then say that we are concerned about fighting homophobia, and heterosexism, and changing attitudes, we're not talking about people being pleasant to us. We're talking about ensuring that the plumber and his assistant aren't standing over our beds with their damn wrenches or knives. Everyone should have safety and freedom of choice. We have the right not to be intimidated in our homes or on the streets because we're Black, or on welfare, or gay.

Jewelle: Right. My lover and I went camping in New Mexico recently. One day we camped on the Rio Grande in a fairly isolated area. We put up our tent and went away for a while. When we returned, there were these guys fishing nearby and it made us really nervous. In fact, we had a long, serious discussion about our mutual terror of being a lesbian couple in an isolated area with these men nearby.

I was especially conscious of us being an interracial couple and how much that might enrage some people.

Barbara: Oh yes, absolutely. Speaking from experience, I think it's easier for two Black women who are lovers to be together publicly than it is for a mixed couple. To me, that's a dead give-away because this is such a completely segregated society. Whenever I had a lover of a different race, I felt that it was like having a sign or a billboard over my head that said: 'These are dykes. Right here.' Because you don't usually see people of different races together in this country, it was almost by definition telling the world that we were lesbians. I think the same is true for inter-racial gay male couples. So, you see, the terror you were feeling was based on fact. Just recently a lesbian was murdered while she and her lover were on the Appalachian trail in Pennsylvania. This is what colours and affects our lives in addition to Howard Beach and Bernhard Goetz.[2]

Jewelle: The guy who murdered the lesbian on the Appalachian trail claimed his defence was that he had been enraged by seeing their blatant lesbianism. He believed he had a right to shoot them because he had been disturbed by their behaviour.

Barbara: What is that defence called? The homophobic panic?

Jewelle: To me, it's equivalent to the Twinkie defence.[3]

Barbara: Yes. There's a term of defence they try to trot out that suggests that the mere existence of gay people is so enraging to some that they are then justified in committing homicide.

Jewelle: It's sort of like saying that because you are scared of the colour black you are justified in running over Black people in Howard Beach.

Barbara: Right. We as a race of people would generally find that kind of thinking ludicrous. Yet there are Black people who would say that those murdered lesbians got what they deserved. I think that some Black men abhor

Black lesbians because we are, by definition, women they are never going to control. I think something snaps in their psyche when they realise that Black lesbians are saying, 'No way. I'm with women and that's that.'

Jewelle: I think it's a psychological thing. Black women are perceived as property and they are the means by which Black men define themselves. It's another way they are like white men. They use female flesh to define themselves. They try to consume us to prove themselves as men because they're afraid to look inside of themselves. The final note about our terror in New Mexico was that it was both a positive and negative thing. It was positive because we refused to give up ground. We decided to stay where we were because we liked the spot. Of course, it meant that I slept with a large rock in my hands and she with her knife open. But I'll tell you, I slept very well and she did too.

Barbara: I'm glad you said that about not giving up ground because as out Black lesbians we have to live and do live with an incredible amount of courage. I've always felt that if anybody tried to physically violate me, that I would do my best to kill them. That's just fact. I'm taller than average. I'm as tall as most men and I don't slouch. When they're looking for people to harass, I feel like they skip me. [*Laughs.*]

Jewelle: I've frequently felt that way too because I'm big. But I think that one of the things that's happening now with the homophobic backlash is that our size and presence enrage them too.

Barbara: That's why self-defence is so important. As people of colour, as lesbians and gay men, we live with potential or actual danger.

Back to the point about courage. I attended a conference several years ago for women organising around poverty and economic issues in the deep South. The Black women who came to the conference were wonderful and they treated me gloriously. As usual, I was out as a lesbian at this conference. Homophobia was the one issue they had not considered as a barrier to women's leadership. Funny thing, they skipped that. [*Laughter.*] But there was a little quorum of white and Black lesbians and we raised the issue. We got up on the stage and read a statement about homophobia. Then we invited other lesbians and people in solidarity with us to stand up. Almost everybody in the room stood up. Later we were talking about the incident in our small groups and a woman said something I'll never forget. She said that what we'd done had taken a lot of courage. And I have never forgotten those words because they came from a woman who was in a position to know the meaning of courage. She knew what it meant because she had been hounded by white bigots all her life. For her to recognise our being out as courage meant a lot to me.

Jewelle: That's a very important point. I think that for those of us in Manhattan, Brooklyn, Albany, we have a certain leeway in being out. We have a diverse women's community that supports us in our efforts to be honest about being lesbians. I find it sad that there is a larger proportion of Black lesbians in small, rural communities who won't and can't come out because they don't have this support. I think they suffer an isolation and even a kind of perversion of their own desires. That's one of the things that Ann Allen Shockley writes about so well – the Black lesbian who is isolated and psychically destroyed because she doesn't have a positive reflection of herself. These are the stories that aren't often told. Such Black lesbians don't get many opportunities to share what is going on for them.

Barbara: Yes. Class is a factor, too.

Jewelle: Certainly. Your whole view about what it means to be lesbian is coloured by whether you were able to get an education – to read different things about the experience.

Barbara: Another point I want to make is that the people who are not out and have the privilege of good education and jobs need to be more accountable. It really bothers me that there are closeted people who are perceived as leaders within the Black community. This is something I find very annoying, because I think they are skating. If they were out on the job or in the community, they would automatically bring together issues that have been counterposed to each other for too long.

Jewelle: Yes. They are skating on our efforts and devotion. It happens all the time. Another thing we need to talk about is religion in the Black community and how it has been such a sustainer in our lives. I find it despicable and a desecration that our spiritual beliefs are perverted and used against Black gay people. Anyone who understands what the spirit of Christianity is supposed to be would never use it against gays.

Barbara: Love thy neighbour as thyself.

Jewelle: Right. Christianity does not say pick and choose which neighbours you're going to love. And any of those biblical quotes that are used against Black gays need to be looked at in the context that that selfsame Bible has been used to depict Blacks as inhuman. Racists use Christianity against Black people and then Black people turn around and use Christianity against gays. It doesn't make any sense to me.

Barbara: We also need to discuss some of the young Black men who are so prominent today in the Hollywood movie and television industry. People like Arsenio Hall, Eddie Murphy, etc. I think they are homophobic to their hearts.

Jewelle: And sexist. I think it's telling that Spike Lee, the most popular Black filmmaker in the country today, includes the rape of a Black woman in his films. Sexism is so pervasive in our community that we don't even think of this as awful. Imagine what it feels like to sit in a movie theatre watching his film *School Daze* in which a Black woman is raped. The so-called Black brothers in the movie

200

are saying, 'Yeah, bone her. Bone her.' And the Black women in the audience are giggling.

Barbara: They were probably giggling because they knew they had to go back home with those kinds of guys. This gets back to the Central Park rape that obsessed and terrorised me so much. The question I was raising at that time is: do men understand that they can kill a woman by raping her? Do they understand that rape is torture and terror for us?

Jewelle: I think that as Black lesbians, in some ways, we are very fortunate. This is because we are in a community that supports us in growing past racism, sexism and homophobia. But as you've said, our heterosexual sisters have to go home with these guys.

Barbara: We have to acknowledge that there are heterosexual Black females who are not putting up with that stuff. There are definitely Black heterosexual feminists who are saying, 'No way. I'm not taking that kind of abuse, negation or suppression.' And as more Black women become feminists, the men are going to have to change. My impression is that there used to be more co-operation between Black men and Black women. Back when lynching was a daily American pastime and the crazed white man was our common enemy, we were not as inclined to lash out against each other as we are today.

For instance, there was an article recently in *Publishers Weekly* about Black writers. The thrust of the piece was that Black male writers are suffering because Black women writers are getting lots of attention. This kind of thinking is based on the scarcity model that says there is only so much approval for Black writers within the mainstream white publishing industry. And that may be true. But there should be infinite approval within a Black context. Everybody who wants to write should write so we can all keep moving on up a little higher.

Jewelle: Can you believe we've had this whole discussion without mentioning *The Color Purple*? To me, the criticism of the book and the film was very much like what happened to Ntozake Shange. People couldn't handle seeing Black women bond, even if it was only on celluloid. So it prompted unbelievable scenarios like grown men sitting at conferences debating whether Alice Walker should have been *allowed* to write *The Color Purple*.

Barbara: What does that say about where we are? And as I've said at exactly those kinds of discussions, if people think *The Color Purple* is an exaggeration of Black women's lives, they should go to any casualty department, battered women's shelter or rape crisis centre in this country. If they did that, they would see that *The Color Purple* is mild, bland and minimal compared to what is actually happening to women and children in this society.

Jewelle: I'd like to close by saying that homophobia is particularly dangerous for Black lesbians because it is so insidious. There have always been acceptable places for gay Black men to retreat and escape from the danger, i.e. the 'choir queen' or the Black gay man who embraces the white gay male community. But as Black gay women, we haven't been interested in removing ourselves from our families or communities because we understand the importance of that connection. The insidiousness of the homophobia lies in the fact that we've been forced to find ways to balance our contact with the community with our need to continue to grow as Black lesbians. We straddle the fence that says we cannot be the uplifters of the race and lesbians at the same time – that's what makes it so dangerous for our emotional health as Black lesbians. But you know, I think that our ability to see the need to keep the family intact is what is going to be our saviour and help preserve the Black community. As lesbians, we have so much to teach the Black community about survival.

Barbara: I'm very glad that you said that about family. One of the myths that's put out about Black lesbians and gay men is that we go into the white gay community and forsake our racial roots. People say that to be lesbian or gay is to be somehow racially denatured. I have real problems with that because that's never been where I was coming from. And that's not the place that the Black lesbians and gays I love, respect and work with are coming from either. We are as Black as anybody ever thought about being. Just because we are committed to passionate and ongoing relationships with members of our own gender does not mean that we are not Black. In fact, the cultural and political leadership of the Black community has always had a very high percentage of lesbian and gay men. Although closeted in many cases, Black lesbians and gays have been central in building our freedom.

Jewelle: I think the political code has always been that you don't bring people out who don't want to come out – you don't force anyone out of the closet. But I think that's changing.

Barbara: [*Laughs.*] I'm delighted, very delighted.

Jewelle: With the way the media works now it's almost impossible to stay closeted. And I don't think people who are out feel as morally obliged to protect the ones who stay in the closet.

Barbara: Especially now that there's AIDS. The ideology that you can just sit back and let a part of your community die off because of homophobia is untenable at this time. There won't be anybody here.

Jewelle: Yes. It's very important that all our voices be heard. Everyone asks why do we have to talk about homophobia? Why can't we be quiet about it? The fact that we have to talk about it means that a lot of people don't want to hear it. And as soon as there's something they don't want to hear, it's very important that we say it. I learned that as a Black person.

Barbara: I'd like to challenge all the non-lesbians to think about what they can do to improve the chances that we'll all be free and sisters.

Notes

1. In response to repeated police harassment, a group of gays rioted at the Stonewall Inn bar in New York in June 1969. The rebellion is considered the start of gay liberation.
2. In December 1984 Bernhard Goetz gunned down four Black youths on a Manhattan subway after alleging they had tried to rob him. In 1987 a gang of white New York teenagers attacked several Black men who had stopped in their Howard Beach neighborhood for pizza. One Black youth was killed by a car as he fled.
3. A defence used by San Francisco Supervisor Dan White in his 1979 trial for the slaying of the city's mayor and a politically powerful and openly gay city supervisor. White's attorney argued that his client's consumption of junk food contributed to his state of diminished capacity.

Therapeutic Bodywork

Sula Thomas Forero

As you read this article notice how you are holding your body? Are you comfortable? Does your seating adequately support your posture? How deeply are you breathing? Could you get into a more comfortable position that supports your ability to breath and your posture? Making adjustments where we can, to the minor discomforts that we feel throughout the day can act as a form of prevention. Our physical discomforts announce that something is not quite right. So many adults experience ongoing tension in their bodies, it is easy to believe that it is just part of being human. Much of our tension is felt within our bodies when our pains are disconnected from our conscious awareness.

Our bodies are the vehicle through which we live our lives; they are an exact physical expression of our deepest feelings, thoughts and emotions. Even our language reveals this fact. For example, most people understand that many of the social pressures that we face can be 'a pain in the neck', or 'hard to stomach'. A great many of us have had to hold down 'back breaking' jobs in conditions that are enough to make 'our blood boil'. Talking about such things helps to 'get it off our chests'. These sayings are not simply poetic metaphors; they are an attempt to describe what is going on beneath our skin: the feeling states and

...at precede physical responses. They hint at the ...nism by which our experiences and responses are pable of adversely affecting our health.

Yet when we go to the average GP with our aches, pains and ills our condition is seldom perceived within the wider context of our entire being and lives. Modern medicine comes near to the acknowledgement of the wider context when it refers to 'psychosomatic' symptoms. The problem is that psychosomatic symptoms are frequently misperceived as existing 'mainly in the mind'. Such an interpretation trivialises our experience and distorts the reality of how our bodies actually function. The implication is that mind and brain are not part of matter. It is not nature that created the divide between mind and matter; the modern medical health paradigm conditioned itself to believe in it.

We have 'thinking', 'feeling' bodies that respond to our entire experience. The ancient health paradigm of natural medicine understands that the fields of the mind, the body, the emotions and energy form an interrelated whole: what exists in one will be reflected in all the others. This is not just a theoretical construct it is inherently practical. When we hold onto processes of thought and emotions through habit and attachment, they become physically manifest in our bodies. When thoughts and emotions become crystallised in the physical body, the energy reflexes that relate to the currents affected, will eventually become unbalanced. The invented split between what goes on in our bodies and minds, has done much to undermine and confuse our understanding of our own bodies. My personal experience of this is one of the things that eventually led me into the field of holistic medicine and therapies.

Thirteen years ago I became ill with chest pain, shortness of breath and irregular heart rhythms. I could barely eat, metabolise food or defecate. My weight dropped; my body struggled to function. I was hospitalised a number of times but no one seemed to understand what was wrong.

I was given two conflicting medical opinions: one that I had a heart condition, the other that the symptoms were psychosomatic and therefore 'all in my mind'. The medication that I was given to treat my 'mind' and my 'heart' did little to help; but being forced to give up my work meant that I had time to myself. This enabled me to get a clearer picture of what was really going on and what I really needed. I had been relentlessly driving myself over the years, disconnected from who I was, or what I needed as a person. I had shut out all the things, past and present, that needed to be healed. The symptoms were my body's way of crying out that it had had enough; that it was time for healing and change. Eventually I healed through my own efforts, the healing process closely paralleled my ability to experience the old hurts out; which then made room for who I was and what I needed.

Not all aberrations are genetic, not all diseases are caused by micro-organisms, not all conditions respond to surgery, drugs or technology. The realisation of this has formed the context for the present popularity of therapeutic bodywork and other forms of natural medicine and therapies.

One of the most overlooked causes of deterioration and ill-health in the body is that of resistance. The aim of therapeutic bodywork is to treat this, which each therapy does in its own unique way. Resistance arises as a result of having a traumatic experience through the body, the senses, the mind and the energy systems. The trauma could be illness; infection; an accident; an injury; a birth trauma; emotional or psychological stress. It seems that when we have not 'completed' a traumatic experience, part of our awareness disassociates from the 'injured' part of the body. This happens as a coping mechanism for that period, but it may remain in place for weeks, months or even years; or until a similar memory triggers the original memory; or until we feel safe enough to discard the protective shield and 'feel' again. The problem is that the shield minimises the amount of energy flow and sensation through the area. The shield will often manifest as some kind of change in the body tissues such as adhesions, tensions, altered circulation, numbness and countless other manifestations. These affect our vitality and aliveness, our ability to make appropriate and healthy choices for ourselves because they disorganise and fragment the system. This is precisely what was happening in my body when I became ill. Removing resistance helps integrate the body, mind and emotions and helps reorganise the body by improving the flow of energy. This often produces or assists in healing.

Our bodies' integrity of prime health and functional efficiency depends not only on our internal chemistry influenced by our thoughts, the nature of the food and drink that we ingest and the air we breathe. It also depends on effective nerve and blood circulation, free of structural and functional obstructions. This is also dependent on the appropriate stimulation and movement of our bodies. When the blood and nerve supply are impaired the body cannot orchestrate its functions in a healthy and organised manner: the nervous system fails to send appropriate commands to different parts of the body. The nutrients carried in the blood and fluid systems cannot adequately nourish the tissues and cells; waste cannot move out of them effectively, which builds septic waste fluids that clog the tissues. This causes further stiffness and pain in the tissues and creates the ideal breeding ground for diseases.

As the fluid systems of blood, hormones and lymph become impaired, the result is either the delivery pressure of the blood has to rise, requiring dangerously increased effort from the heart and capillaries; or the body tissues have to make do with a lower volume of fluids. Considering that the circulatory system of the body carries every element that our cells depend on for their productivity and survival and that it carries away all of their metabolic waste, it becomes easier to see how the body is adversely affected by chronic tension/resistance. The waste products of chronic tension create what is termed 'gluing' of our body tissues. Old wastes form acids that actually stick together muscles and body tissues that were designed to glide freely over one another.

This can make us feel profoundly uncomfortable within our own bodies. The body begins to feel stiff, tight and cramped, as if it doesn't 'fit well' any more and in fact it doesn't because the tissues are being pulled, tightened and 'hitched up' so that the body becomes restricted. Movements then begin to feel heavy and laboured as our muscles have the added burden of dragging neighbouring muscle groups along that were never intended to move together. The gluing creates the thickenings, shortenings and restrictions associated with ageing, repeated strain and poorly healed injuries. Experiencing this we exclaim, 'My body is becoming stiff because I am getting old', when more often than not, it would be more accurate to say 'My body is stiff and painful due to inadequate movement and an accumulation of unresolved stresses'. Ageing is, to a large degree, the sum total of stressors that we have accumulated throughout a lifetime; but ageing does not have to be a gradual decline towards illness and infirmity. Bodywork can help to keep our body tissue supple, bouncy and resilient throughout a lifetime. Often, the tighter our bodies become, the less awareness they are capable of; subsequently the less able we are to sense what our bodies are actually experiencing, until the tension and resistance pops into our conscious awareness as pain and discomfort.

Our bodies learn to take on a form/structure that they feel most 'comfortable' with, even though it may be one of discomfort, because our minds identify with that form on a very deep level. The skill therefore, in many forms of therapeutic bodywork, is in being able to meet a person where they are, with openness, respect and clear intention; observing how the body wishes to change and then following that. The body knows its own healing process and this becomes evident when you start massaging or manipulating restricted body tissues; and they begin to move into 'the right place'. Often you can feel this underneath your fingers, and following this movement will help create changes in the body that are in tune with everything else that is going on for that person. Therapeutic bodywork can assist us in getting to know our own bodies. 'Hands-on' bodywork is a concrete and practical way of reinforcing the interrelationships of our body systems and our minds in a very direct way. It can help us to more readily understand what we are made of, to more accurately assess our condition and reveal to us how we gain freedom from the restrictions that lock us into self-perpetuating cycles of stress and exhaustion. Stress and tension are kept 'alive' mainly through our nervous systems.

When any of the nerve centres in our body are in a state of hyperactivity they will attempt to discharge the excess energy to other organs or structures such as the musco-skeletal system, the stomach or the lungs; the stress thus gets referred. Over the years therapeutic bodywork has been one of the most effective ways through which I have been able to heal and recover my health. The body helps the mind to heal and the mind helps the body; bodywork helps both levels to integrate healing. In this way, talking therapy such as counselling or psychotherapy, pairs well with bodywork. Looking back, I can see how my own experiences helped shape my interest in health-related studies and eventually bodywork.

I have been studying therapeutic bodywork for the last seven years, and for the last five I have worked in this field both in private practice and as part of a multi-disciplinary team within the health service. Practice and study have helped to enhance my understanding of the body and to broaden the scope of my work. The main disciplines I practise are therapeutic massage and reflexology. These work by balancing the three aspects of the nervous system which are related to the three poles of energy expression within the body. I also practise cranio-sacral therapy, a diagnostic and therapeutic way of assisting the body's core energy. The fourth discipline I practise is Zen-therapy, a synthesis of bodywork methods developed over many years by Dub Leigh from the USA. The core of Zentherapy involves structural integration which releases the body from life long accumulations of pain and tensions that build up in our muscles and myo-fascial system. Fascia is the tough fibro-elastic tissue which connects, integrates and supports our body structure and function. Fascia covers and supports every muscle organ and vessel of the human body. It is the integrating tissue of the body, as it is one interconnecting sheet that wraps around every single body part and is continuous from the top of our heads to the bottom of our feet. In this way, a restriction or imbalance in one area will not only upset the structural integrity and balance of the body, but can also affect the internal health-regulating processes. Zentherapy systematically realigns the muscles and myo-fascial system so that gravity assists rather than burdens the structural integrity of the body. This is achieved through penetrating manipulation of the body and assisting the flow of vital energy. It also involves re-education of bodily use and movement, much of which arises from the work of Feldenkrais (see below).

The field of bodywork is vast and covers many different traditions, including therapeutic massage, holistic massage, shiatsu, reflexology, polarity therapy, aromatherapy, acupuncture, cranio-sacral therapy, kinesiology, osteopathy, chiropractice, rolfing (the original method of structural integration developed by the late Dr Ida P. Rolf, USA), the Alexander technique and the Feldenkrais method. The Feldenkrais method was developed by the late Dr Moshe Feldenkrais. It consists of what are called 'awareness through movement' exercises and 'functional integration', both of which help people correct the neuro-muscular limitations that contribute to stress and inability to accomplish goals. All of these methods are used in health assessment and maintenance; in prevention and healing. Many bodywork practices originate in antiquity and are based on principles used in traditional folk medicine, especially in the ancient cultures of Africa, India and China, which are rich in such types of medicine. In the West today such practices are often referred to as 'alternative' or 'complementary', but they are really the ancient foundations of medicinal practice, which have survived through thousands of years of use and development. For many black women traditional/natural medicine, especially in Africa, the Caribbean and Brazil, is an integral part of health care, and has survived particularly within the form of herbal knowledge, wisdom and lore. Many of our mothers, grandmothers and great-grandmothers had great herbal knowledge; my maternal great-grandmother from Sierra Leone was one such woman.

Ancient traditions laid the foundations for some of the more recent developments in natural medicine and bodywork today. Reflexology, a therapy based on stimulation of the pressure points of the hands and feet, comes from a method that originated in ancient Egypt. The earliest documentation of reflexology was unearthed around 233 BC in the physician's tomb of Ankmahor at Saqqarain Egypt.[1] What is known as osteopathy today is a method developed from the practice of 'bone-setting'. In ancient Egypt bone-setters were renowned for their skill, and bone-setters form a part of traditional medicine in most parts of Africa, for example Liberia, Zimbabwe and Nigeria. Swedish massage, a popular form of massage in Europe and America, was pioneered at the beginning of this century by a Swede, Per Henrik Ling, who developed the method by synthesising knowledge from the fields of gymnastics, physiology and Egyptian, Roman and Greek massage.

One form of massage common to African and Caribbean cultures is baby massage, the benefits of which are now becoming more widely appreciated in the West. Massage of the newborn child can be invaluable to the early years of a child's development. The effect of therapeutic touch is so powerful that newborn mammals, including humans, can die, if they are deprived of touch. This was happening in the orphanages of Europe and America in the early part of this century until investigations discovered the underlying cause of the 99 per cent infant mortality rates of abandoned infants who were dying within one year of admission.[2] A large number of physical and emotional disturbances can result if the amount of touch in the early years of a child's development is inadequate or if the touch received is abusive. Massage facilitates the mother–child bonding process and is a way of putting information into the body at a very basic level. The more detailed and clear this 'information', the more raw data the brain has to assemble an accurate image of itself which helps it to track, stimulate and organise its own functions. It helps 'fine-tune' the body–brain connection, which heightens the body's self-regulatory and self-healing capacity. This occurs via the stimulation of the sensory nerve endings in the skin that feed back information to the deepest levels of the body and brain. Paediatric research shows that premature babies progress far more rapidly when regularly massaged[3]

Many older black women whom I have treated recall, from 'back home', massaging their newborns, or being massaged themselves as children. Many women who massage their babies say they find that their babies sleep and feed better and that it helps prevent and treat problems such as wind, indigestion, constipation and colic. Massage can be used throughout life as a form of preventative and curative treatment to help restore and maintain health. Some women use massage as part of their prenatal healthcare; one of the more common reasons that women seek massage at this time is that it nurtures their bodies through the process of change. It helps resolve stress, increases stamina, decreases water retention, eases back pain, enhances the overall well-being of mother and child and can be very useful during labour. Following the birth, massage can be used to help relax and support the mother and to support the body's efforts towards regeneration and healing. Massage is one of the most basic yet powerful forms of bodywork, and is relatively easily learnt. A good friend of mine taught her children to massage themselves and each other from an early age. Now when they have a minor ailment such as a headache or stomach ache, they know that stimulating certain parts of the body can help to relieve these and that they do not always have to resort to using pills. It is also a good way of teaching them to care for themselves and others.

When I started out practising massage I found that there was a great demand for massage amongst black women in the African and Caribbean communities. Seeing how women were responding to massage instigated my interest to learn more about bodywork. Some of the most common benefits that women report are: an easing or resolution of pain, improved sleep and concentration, greater calm and available energy. Greater ease and comfort in the body often comes about, and women generally become less vulnerable to stress. If we do not resolve stress we become vulnerable to burnout. I have come across many black women who use their wills to keep on going, even after the point of exhaustion, due to the pressures we face to be strong and coping in this society. Some of the commonest complaints I have observed when working with black women in our communities are back, neck and shoulder pain; tiredness, depression, high blood pressure, chest pain or discomfort, exhaustion and disconnection from the body.

The conventional approach to most of these, more often than not, is to prescribe medication. Quite often drugs offer temporary relief by masking or alleviating the symptoms. Analgesics, for example, perform one valuable service: they block pain signals. The problem is that pain is a warning of imbalance within the body; the injured part is sending electrical and chemical messages through the nervous system where the pain is interpreted. Masking pain, therefore, is a bit like taking the batteries out of the warning light. The underlying cause of the pain remains undealt with, therefore unhealed. In less common, severe cases back problems can be caused by a problem such as gallstones, kidney problems or gynaecological dysfunction. If you experience back pain with weakness in the legs or have trouble urinating, take medical advice immediately. Back problems are often treated with limited success as a local problem, when most back pain is a symptom of an imbalance in the way the upper body balances on the pelvis and legs. Let's consider lower back pain. The lower back is where the major muscle groups and sheaths meet to form the midsection of the body. It is also our centre of gravity and is therefore a potential source of great compression. As it is also our centre of gravity, the lower back is extremely vulnerable to forces of resistance coming from anywhere else in the body. A lower back problem, therefore is not necessarily originating in your back. Back pain is mainly due to structural and functional disorganisations, although other influencing factors may be involved.

In holistic medicine or therapy there are three elements that constitute the entire human organism and its functions: the physical/structural, mental/emotional and nutritional/chemical. These determine our health and the movement and flow of the electrical energy circuits in our bodies. Our health and energy circuits can in turn be interrupted by nutritional, mental and physical influences. Faulty nutrition can contribute to and exacerbate back pain. This could be a simple lack of water or a more complex pattern of nutritional deficiency. If we are low in the nutrients that support and nourish our body tissues, imbalances within them can occur. As the biochemistry of muscular contractions requires large amounts of calcium, magnesium and other nutrients; if our muscles are tightly contracted the body begins to be stripped of these vital nutrients. Stress, physical trauma and poor bodily mechanics such as poor seating or bedding, lack of exercise and the extra strain that can be imposed due to pregnancy or being overweight can also be the cause of back pain. Research shows that in parts of Africa where women squat rather than sit and are generally active, there is little incidence of back trouble, and X-rays of the spine show no sign of the degeneration you would expect to see in people from the West.[4]

When black women came to Britain in the 1950s and 1960s the sociopolitical and economic climate meant that many ended up in some of the most physically taxing backbreaking jobs. I know of many black women who have sustained mechanical strains or injury during heavy labour. Many of these women have not received appropriate and effective treatment. Women's high-heeled footwear also frequently cause or contribute to back pain, as they throw the weight of the upper body forwards so that the lower body structures have to overly contract in an attempt to rebalance the weight.

The little habits we adopt can also throw the body out of alignment: form follows function and function follows form. Many of us place more of our body weight on one leg in standing and walking; a lot of us have difficulty separating eye movements from neck movements. Although very subtle, these small functional habits build contractions and compensations in our bodies. On a psycho-emotional level, 'holding back' our inner urges, drives and creativity can build up a lot of tension in our backs. Another psycho-emotional issue is that of support. Feeling an absence of psychological and emotional support, our back or other muscles may become rigid in an attempt to create the illusion of the support we require. Sometimes our bodies may take the opposite stance, that of collapsing. All of these relationships are circular not linear. Different influences provoke and reflect others. Therapeutic bodywork has much to teach us about relationship.

Recently I worked with a woman who complained of lower back pain, as well as digestive disturbances and fatigue. This coexistence of symptoms is common, when the body sets itself in a dysfunctional posture; this can cramp the internal structures and organs and affect the way in which they function. Tension almost always accompanies fatigue, as tension squanders an enormous amount of our available energy. When undergoing regular bodywork some symptoms are given a chance to improve or heal themselves as the body becomes more flowing and organised. Chronic muscle contractions, depending on their location can give rise to disturbances of the respiratory, digestive, urogenital, eliminative or reproductive organs. Constipation, menstrual cramps and haemorrhoids can arise from chronically contracted tissues surrounding the trunk and pelvic region.

In the case of some forms of haemorrhoids, contractions of muscle groups including the perineal muscle, gives rise to chronic contraction of the anus, creating intolerable pressure in the anal sphincter. During defecation the anus cannot relax, causing great pressure to the blood vessels and surrounding tissues, in forcing the contents of the anus out of the body. The conventional treatment is often injections to shrink the haemorrhoids or surgery to remove them. However I have found that releasing the tension and balancing the muscle groups will often spontaneously correct the condition. I experienced this myself through receiving deep-tissue bodywork. These are all examples of why the treatment of back pain with medication does not usually address the primary causes. Successful treatment may mean looking at a number of different factors together, and making changes accordingly. A combination of osteopathy and massage may be successful in the treatment of much back pain.

The high incidence of hypertension in black people in Britain and the USA gives cause for concern, since high blood pressure is known to be closely linked to heart disease. The treatment for hypertension is usually drugs, and the doctor's advise that the patient should relax. The name hints at one of hypertension's contributory causes, that is, being in a state of 'hyper' (excessive) tension. Unfortunately conditions in this society frequently give us much to be hypertense about: concerns about housing, employment, work, redundancy, money, our own safety and that of our children, as well as the overt and covert racial hostility we face.

It is well known that massage helps reduce blood pressure.[5] When teaching massage skills to nurses some years ago, I asked them to monitor blood pressure before and after every massage. What we found was that every subject's blood pressure dropped, except those who had low blood pressure. After a massage most people's blood pressure will fall, although it is also true it may then rise again. Blood pressure tends to vary throughout the day, going up when we are excited and falling when we are relaxed. One of the things that may be significant in keeping it high is chronically contracted muscle tissue. Deep massage and other forms of bodywork that penetrate the deeper levels are more likely to have a stabilising influence on blood pressure.

Some of the black women I have worked with have suffered chronically contracted chests. With a tight chest the intercostal muscles between the ribs are often jammed. The relationship between the state of the tissues and the rhythms of the heart and breathing is a very direct one. Tight body tissues alter the breath wave, making it flow less well than it should. When the breath cycle is impaired, the heart has to work harder; when the heart lacks energy, then breathing works to make up the difference. When the energy that breath was intended to provide does not flow freely, then rigidity starts to spread through the body tissues. An article in *The Sunday Times* in October 1992, 'Take a deep breath', considered these relationships in a new approach to heart disease. This approach, which is being investigated by top British cardiologist Dr Peter Nixon, places the main emphasis on the breathing pattern. Although his colleagues disagree he believes that beyond the conventional risk factors such as hypertension, high cholesterol and smoking that 'hyperventilation' or over-breathing plays a more fundamental role in generating heart problems. Hyperventilation commonly occurs when we are stressed and tense. Breath that is shallow, irregular and rapid causes the blood to become saturated with oxygen and low in carbon dioxide, which alters the acid alkaline balance of the body with far reaching effect. It triggers the body's fight or flight mechanisms, which in turn lead to a breach of the body's homoeostatic safety mechanisms. The alkaline state increases the calcium content of the heart cells, causing a stiffening of heart tissue. It makes blood vessels constrict, with a rising increase in the pressure.

This makes perfect sense to me. In bodywork one of the most effective ways of enabling a person to breathe more freely is to release any body tissues that are involved in restraining the breath wave. Merely instructing someone with a chronically restricted chest, neck and lower body to 'breathe deeply' will not produce lasting results if their body form prevents sustained deep breathing. I have found that during bodywork, once a person's stomach, chest and diaphragm have softened and opened, very often the whole body will begin to stream with aliveness, energy and sensation, because when these structures release it is like unblocking an energetic dam. On the emotional level, the chest is a place where we hold back many of our feelings: it is an area that we sometimes close up to protect. It is also one of the places where we experience the urge to reach out and make contact. Sometimes we may have conflict between the two, but releasing the chest can literally help to open up our emotional heart.

Static contraction of muscle tissues can raise blood pressure; this is what happens in isometric exercise and when the body is in chronic tension. Isometric exercise is known to cause a sharp rise in blood pressure.[6] After isometric contractions, blood pressure can rise by as much as 50 per cent.[7] Even simple static contraction of the arm, if sustained, will elevate blood pressure by 10– 20 mmHg.[8] 'Essential' hypertension is a medical term for hypertension which has no 'known' cause such as kidney dysfunction. There are many hypotheses as to the cause of hypertension, including genetic and dietary considerations. Although stress is now being given more emphasis as a major factor in illness and disease, we still hear little about the actual physiology of stress and its exact effects within our bodies. The vast majority of Western trained doctors are not trained to view the relationships of structural, functional and energetic balances and their relationship to stress in the way many bodywork practitioners are trained to.

As a result they could be missing a vital link in understanding the cause of essential hypertension and countless other conditions. Although not commonly referred to in Western medical practice, there exists masses of research, conducted all over the world, particularly within the field of manipulative therapies and osteopathic medicine that reveal these relationships quite clearly. All disciplines need to work together so that we do not have gaps in our health care. Health maintenance and preventive treatment should be just as important as, if not more important than, the present emphasis on treating illness and disease. Our health system is in crisis and one of the things that is badly needed is safer, cheaper, less intrusive forms of care and a deeper understanding of the many facets that influence human health and disease. We are spiritual as well as material beings and care of the soul is missing from present day medicine. It is well known that the best GPs or healers are not those who merely possess technical know-how, but those who are sensitive and intuitive and make the closest and most compassionate contact with their patients.

If the true concerns and objectives of the health service is people's health, there is no reason why holistic and conventional medicine cannot coexist. Modern medical practitioners are already stretched beyond their limits. If the two systems work together it could make the difference between people having to struggle on with countless untreated discomforts and ailments, and recovery as a result of appropriate and effective treatment. No one system has the answer, each has part of the answer. Multi-disciplinary approaches can produce remarkable results. We need choice. Through choice we have wider options and through options we learn what works for us and what doesn't.

In 1991 when legislation gave GPs the option of managing the funds of their own practices, it was agreed that they could employ complementary therapists. If you are registered at one of these practices and feel you would benefit from bodywork or any other form of complementary medicine or therapy, it is worth asking. The more people make their needs for wider options in health care known, the more chance there is of change being brought about.

If you decide you would like to have professional bodywork, the first thing is to establish your particular need.
This might be general relaxation and stress reduction, or a
specific complaint that needs attention. If you telephone or
visit a centre most practitioners and therapists will be happy
to discuss whether their discipline is likely to suit your
needs. Word of mouth or some women's centres can be a
good way of finding a practitioner. There are a growing
number of black women practitioners and therapists who
offer bodywork.

As bodywork involves a certain degree of intimacy, the
chemistry and communication between you and the
practitioner needs to be right. You should be able to
express what does or doesn't feel comfortable to you.
When you find a practitioner you may want to know what
their qualifications are and what these mean. Buying a
book on the subject may help. One of the best is *The
Complementary Health Guide* edited by Amanda Chambers.[9]
Some practitioners and centres have a sliding scale of fees;
others don't. Some community based organisations who
do, are listed at the end of this book.

Notes

1. I. Dougans with S. Ellis, *The Art of Reflexology (A Step-by-Step
   Guide)*, Element Books Ltd , Shaftesbury, Dorset 1992, p. 10.
2. D. Juhan, *A Handbook for Bodywork, Job's Body*, Station Hill Press,
   New York, 1987, pp. 43–44.
3. L. Lidell, *The Book of Massage (The Complete Step-by-Step Guide to
   Eastern and Western Techniques)*, Edbury Press, London, 1985,
   p. 154.
4. S. Moore, *Chiropractic*, (Alternative Health Series), Optima
   Books, London, 1988, p. 93.
5. L. Hodgkinson, 'Hands on Treatment,' *The Sunday Times*,
   25.10.92.
6. T. Hanna, *Somatics (Re-awakening the Mind's Control of Movement,
   Flexibility & Health)*, Addison-Wesley Publishing Co. Inc., New
   York, 1991, p. 73.

7. Ibid.
8. L. Chartow, *Soft-Tissue Manipulation*, Thorsons Publishing, Northamptonshire, 1988, p. 17.
9. A. Chambers, *The Complementary Health Guide*, English Countryside Publications, Colchester, Essex, 1993.

Prescriptions of Root Doctors

Zora Neale Hurston

In 1935 Hurston published Mules and Men, *a vibrant and
magical collection of black folklore she had gathered in the
South. The following excerpt from the book is an invaluable
contribution to our heritage and our understanding of traditional
black folk medicine.*

Folk medicine is practised by a great number of persons.
On the 'job', that is, in the sawmill camps, the turpentine
stills, mining camps and among the lowly generally,
doctors are not generally called to prescribe for illnesses,
certainly, nor for the social diseases. Nearly all of the
conjure doctors practise 'roots', but some of the root
doctors are not hoodoo doctors. One of these latter at
Bogaloosa, Louisiana, and one at Bartow, Florida, enjoy a
huge patronage. They make medicine only, and white and
coloured swarm about them claiming cures.

The following are some prescriptions gathered here and
there in Florida, Alabama and Louisiana:

Bladder trouble
One pint of boiling water, two tablespoons of flax seed,
two tablespoons of cream of tartar. Drink half a glass in the
morning and half at night.

Fistula

Sweet gum bark and mullen cooked down with lard. Make a salve.

Rheumatism

Take mullen leaves (five or six) and steep in one quart of water. Drink three to four wineglasses a day.

Swelling

Oil of white rose (15 cents), oil of lavender (15 cents), Jockey Club (15 cents), Japanese honeysuckle (15 cents). Rub.

Blindness

(a) Slate dust and pulverised sugar. Blow in the eyes. (It must be finely pulverised to remove film.)
(b) Get somebody to catch a catfish. Get the gall and put it in a bottle. Drop one drop in each eye. Cut the skin off. It gives the sight a free look.

Lockjaw

(a) Draw out the nail. Beat the wound and squeeze out all the blood possible. Then take a piece of fat bacon, some tobacco and a penny and tie it on the wound.
(b) Draw out the nail and drive it in a green tree on the sunrise side, and the place will heal.

Flooding★

One grated nutmeg, pinch of alum in a quart of water (cooked). Take half a glass three times daily.

Sick at stomach

Make a tea of parched rice and bay leaves (six). Give a cup at a time. Drink no other water.

★Menstruation.

Live things in stomach (fits)

Take a silver quarter with a woman's head on it. Stand her on her head and file it in one-half cup of sweet milk. Add nine parts of garlic. Boil and give to drink after straining.

Medicine to purge

Jack of War tea, one tablespoon to a cup of water with a pinch of soda after it is ready to drink.

Loss of mind

Sheep weed leaves, bay leaf, sarsaparilla root. Take the bark and cut it all up fine. Make a tea. Take one tablespoon and put in two cups of water and strain and sweeten. You drink some and give some to patient.

Put a fig leaf and poison oak in shoe. (Get fig leaves off a tree that hasn't borne fruit. Stem them so that nobody will know.)

To make a tonic

One quart of wine, three pinches of raw rice, three dusts of cinnamon (about one heaped teaspoon), five small pieces of the hull of pomegranate about the size of a fingernail, five tablespoons of sugar. Let it come to a boil, set one half-hour and strain. Dose: one tablespoon.

(When the pomegranate is in season, gather all the hulls you can for use at other times in the year.)

Breaking the Cycle of Abuse:
Getting to the Root of Self-Defence

Khaleghl Quinn

Each of us is born with a unique beauty – a unique set of gifts to discover and offer the world. This unique code is reflected in our individual features. Take a closer look and you'll find these features to be a mixture of our ancestry, the influence of cultures in our background and the environment in which we habitually find ourselves. Though these parameters may provide the contextual framework for what we are, they pale in the face of who we are and who we may become.

There are many political and social statements that I could make about being a black woman and particularly, a woman of many colours. Much of what I would like to emphasise has already been spoken and indeed well documented. So I would like to share with you some of the fruits of my professional research on a personal level. The past twenty-three years I have channelled my energies into the arena of martial arts psychology and self-defence. This is because I feel they are relevant tools for gaining the confidence required in the quest for living more of our potential. The physical and academic training of these years has afforded and continues to afford me the luxury of looking into the more subtle, yet deeply essential aspects of self-defence. My aim is to expose something that has already been proven empirically by the people, especially women, who have successfully defended themselves in dangerous situations: that self-defence is 90 per cent attitude, based on strong self-esteem and 10 per cent effective physical back-up. The physical knowledge reinforces confidence but is not necessarily the source of it. I have found inner strength to be the source of confidence. Inner strength gives us a sense of our strengths and vulnerabilities. There is acceptance of both – an increasingly working sense of how one can be used to feed the other. Such is the principle of the Eastern concept of yin and yang, or our receptive and active natures. When we are aware of being open and receptive we absorb strength, which leads to being active and even to leadership ability. When we are aware of the limitations of the quality of action that we can make at a given time we can sit back, rest and receive again. When there is room inside us for both these parts, we break through stress and learn to recycle our vital energies. Our strength is resilient. We have choice, and choice is power. It is exactly this sense of choice that I invite you to explore here. Having choice in the simple events of our lives is what builds confidence. As songwriter Holly Near says: 'Linger on the details, the parts that reflect the change. There lies revolution – our everyday lives, the changes inside become our political songs.'

When we create space and time in our lives to think, we have more choice. This is how and why we become proficient at anything, whether dancing, typing, being a parent or brushing our teeth. When we don't feel safe to construct this time and space in our lives to meet our needs we become fertile ground for stress and put other people's needs above our own. In the extreme situation of attack, the degree of our love for ourselves, or *self-esteem, is the crucial motivating factor for fighting back even if that means picking our noses in the face of an attacker in order to put him off.* There are many more subtle forms of attack in our daily lives. These may be the way we relate to the many people we love; the stress of coping with challenges and crises; and the abusive voices we allow to breed within our minds and emotions.

Let us now look at the roots of abuse. Abuse is the direct opposite of self-esteem. By shedding light on these often anonymous, erosive forces within and without we may increase our available energy for self-esteem and self-realisation. Through this awareness we may then find ways to constructively transform our lives, so that the choices we make can become even more fulfilling. It is through this awareness, this inner light, that we may formulate reserves of strength to break through oppressive situations – in our unique ways – in our own timing.

GETTING TO THE ROOT OF SELF-DEFENCE

Our bodies are a grounded physical boundary. They keep what is emotionally appropriate for us separate from what is appropriate for others. We look and sometimes feel different from others, encouraging others to compare themselves to us, or rebelling anarchistically. When our comparisons result in feelings of inferiority or superiority we become unbalanced and lose touch with our individual sense of worth. Whatever the reasons, the loss or gain in self-worth provides the lens through which we approach our daily interactions. An attitude or perspective is developed as a result and we lose the use of our bodies as a grounded physical boundary.

The act of abuse is a response to vulnerability. It is a double-sided coin. On one side of the coin, when loss of self-esteem becomes a ruling motivator in our lives we leave ourselves open to mental, emotional and physical abuse. On the other side, we react by abusing others, because any confrontation with our own weaknesses seems unbearable. As a consequence, the abused learns to remain absorbed in her or his weaknesses; the abuser 'acts out' from fear that their weaknesses will be discovered. In both cases there is an inherent weakening of character. The whole person, complete with their unique set of interests and responses, is eclipsed in this displaced persona. Confidence breaks down as feelings of vulnerability overwhelm and erode the sense of capability we normally build up from birth.

GIVING UP THE LUXURY OF BEING WEAK

This creates an imbalance of force which limits a person's ability to utilise their personal power in a constructive way in the world. Children are particularly susceptible when their immediate environment is sullied by adults, in the home or the school, who occupy one or both sides of the coin of abuse. Abusive adults were once children, and so the cycle persists. **For many of us this inherited cycle of abuse means 'giving up the luxury of being weak'.** I see abuse in terms of the bully and the bullied. This manifests itself, on the one hand, in the spectrum of abuse we are likely to encounter from others within our lifetime; but it also occurs as an insidious, omnipresent bully lurking inside ourselves – a bully we may unwittingly have inherited from our parents, and they from theirs.

A MISCARRIAGE OF BALANCE

In the self-defence world the notion of the bully and the bullied or the attacker and victim is symbiotic with the miscarriage of the balance of power, that is, they are interconnected. Once exposed, this syndrome is capable of bringing about greater potential within each one of us. The need for self-defence is a direct response to the victim/attacker syndrome. **Healing begins with the recognition of the abuser and the abused inside us**. Each of us has had both feelings at some time or another. The seeds of abuse lie within such actions as when, for example, we put ourselves down for no apparent reason, or when we habitually feel the need to put others down in order to feel better about our own problems.

The chronic bully is someone who has learned to suppress any notion of vulnerability or weakness – often in the face of violence inflicted on them. This suppression creates a posture that alienates the bully from his or her more sensitive emotions such as fear, sadness and feelings related to being vulnerable, and therefore from a sense of wholeness and balance. Given habitual suppression, this convoluted volcanic emotion can only be released by acting it out on a likely target, that is on one who has taken on the posture of a chronic victim. Instead of developing constructive assertiveness as a solution to helplessness experienced during vulnerable times, the bully seeks balance outside him/herself, hence the link to the victim. Energetically, this person's energy field is very spiky, jutting out mainly from the chest, jaw and head.

Conversely, the chronic victim is someone who has learned to accept being helpless in relation to others and to life's circumstances and events. A defensive physical, mental and emotional posture develops. Within the shell of this posture the person feels impotent to direct their power outward to effect change within their immediate environment. The only apparent solution (albeit subconscious) is to implode any feelings of potency, turning energy inwards. This inverted energy flow is destructive and leads to self-abuse. It nevertheless continues to recycle, giving a false sense of balance. On an energetic level it is like a bunch of arrows being sucked into a vacuum. This implosion acts as a magnet for any lurking abuser who wants to fulfil his or her fantasy of being less vulnerable and in control.

GUILT – A DISGUISE FOR ATONEMENT

The transmutation of abuse is a complicated issue. Within the arena of the self this syndrome may be acted out when the person feels victimised or embarrassed in any way, for appearing to be vulnerable. This state of imbalance creates discomfort, and once we begin to become aware of it another problem arises – guilt or remorse. We must recognise the guilt as a disguise for atonement. We can utilise guilt as a signal in the process of healing and in the short term as a springboard out of the victim/attacker trap, but we should not think of it as a real step out of it. In fact, it consumes our power to transmute the weakness into more balance and inner strength.

THE POWER TO TRANSFORM

Real transformation can occur when the individual reclaims their mind/body/emotion connection, and programs it to achieve power without doing this at the expense of others. Following are some exercises which help to promote this process. In the first exercise, you may quickly access your mind/body/emotion connection to make it work for you in a healthier way. Increasing the vital energy in your body and your ability to move stagnant energy may help you realise or remember this power you have over yourself. When we focus on ourselves rather than on others, to effect change, 90 per cent of our problems disappear.

In the second exercise you will remember how you are capable of changing your immediate perspective, the way

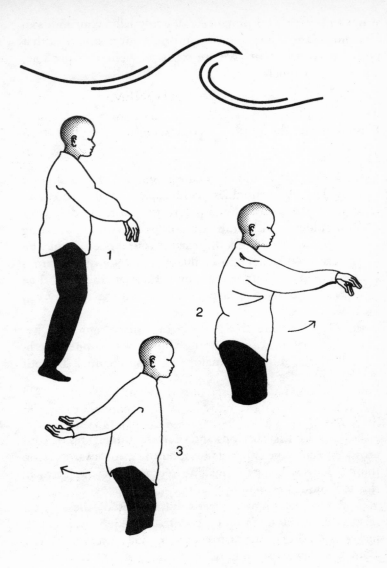

The pump

you set up your environment and, eventually, your lifestyle. The aim of this exercise is to reinforce your memory of that power or your intent. We are what we believe *is* possible, and it does happen.

First exercise: the pump

Preparation

   (a) Stance. Set a solid foundation. Stand with legs slightly wider than shoulder-width apart. Make sure the power base of your pelvis is secure under your shoulders with the tip of your spine pointing downwards toward the earth. Your knees should be comfortably bent to facilitate a springy quality from the top of your pelvis down through the legs. The body should be relaxed and open so that energy can flow freely.

   (b) Now be sure that the tip of your tongue touches the roof of your mouth behind your upper teeth. This will unite the major yin/yang channels in your body.

Technique

   1. Sensitise first the tops and then the undersides of your arms, especially your wrists by focusing your awareness on them. They will be the leading segment of your arms in this technique.

   2. After you have effectively sensitised these areas raise your wrist in front of you to shoulder level *and no higher*. (Raising your arms higher will disconnect you from the power of your belly centre, *tantien*.) Initiate the movement from the centre point of your lower belly. Feel the fullness of this movement as a wave at full crest. This is the upward swing. It pulls the energy up the backs

of your legs along your spine to the top of your head. Hold the fullness for three seconds initially, creating a suspension effect before going to the next half of the technique. The suspension time (quiet time) is of utmost importance in movement meditation sequences, because it is within this expression of intention that the *chi* or vital mind/body energy flows in, bringing insight and illumination.

3. Allow the fullness of the upward swing to be the initiating point of the next motion: the downwards and back swing. The downwards swing allows the *chi* to cascade down into the front of your body, flushing out stagnant energy and sending it into the earth to compost. (When this energy is in the Earth it effectively transforms into more vital energy.) To achieve this next part allow the sensitivity of the underside of the forearms to lead you. Go as far behind your back as you can (without strain) and as high up. The higher up you raise your arms, the more elasticity you will give to your pectoral region, back and shoulders. (This is a very important area. It is the foundation for projecting your love and creativity out into the world, much as the strength and elasticity of the legs are bioenergetically supportive of creating an inner climate of connectedness and confidence.)

This exercise enables you to experience the flow of energy within your body as if it were a wave. Waves are created by opposing forces acting upon the same entity. Celestial attraction and water currents force the ocean upwards, and the earth's gravity brings it crashing back down. In the course of our daily lives, we are faced with a myriad of opposing factions. We are constantly making decisions, choosing options. How we respond to this chaos of opposing forces creates the flow of our days.

The ocean has its own rhythm just as your body does. Feelings of expansion/contraction, tension/relaxation and filling/emptying are often experienced internally as the body pump is being performed. The expansion/ contraction feeling of the body pump is an expression of space: expansion opens up space, contraction shrinks it. Although we are not always conscious of it, expansion and contraction are going on constantly in our bodies. Our hearts and lungs experience this dynamic with each breath, each heartbeat.

On an attitudinal level this relates to how we perceive possibilities in our lives. Have you ever had a day when you felt very closed off, as if almost every facet of your life was somehow stagnant and unsatisfying, and it seemed as if there was very little likelihood that things would ever change? Then, just a few days later everything seems to have opened up, the world seems brighter, the possibility for change is right there in front of you. Some people look upon a piece of paper as just an empty sheet. Others see it as a wealth of possibilities: a poem to be written, a picture not yet drawn, a paper aeroplane to be flown.

Tension and relaxation are two facets of the pump energy which we perceive fairly easily with our five senses. Having experienced the reality of the concepts and the effects of the pump technique, we are now equipped to integrate its value – its meaning. It is at this level that we improve the quality of our life.

The pump shows me that there is a difference between 'knowing' and 'understanding'. The pump is about taking something in, changing it, and then putting it out. We take in knowledge, and it mixes with what's already inside us. This blending can sometimes produce a by-product called wisdom. When we base our actions upon the wisdom inside us, then we show that we do indeed 'understand'.

When we actively tune in and feel the sensation of our heart pumping, we are connected with our feet, our heads, and the pulse of all humanity. Even though our hearts may beat at different rates, the fact that they are all indeed beating establishes common ground. From this platform we may delve deeper to feel our connection with nature – with all living things, animate and inanimate. This delving attitude affords us sensitivity to the forces of life which resonate at different unique rhythms within each individual entity. At this level we hear the symphony of life.

Second exercise: changing your perspective

The following exercise will give you a clear and immediate sense that how you program yourself creates a certain climate of activity.

Exercise A

Without altering the normal position of your head, imagine that the roof of your mouth is closer to the ground than it is to the ceiling. (If you prefer, you can refer to your nose instead.) Walk around with this perspective for three minutes and notice the following:

(a) How are you breathing?
(b) What are you able to see, hear, smell and taste?
(c) What is your general feeling, your mood?
(d) How do you feel towards others in general and towards those in your immediate environment?
(e) What is the pace of your walk?
(f) If someone walked into the room and offered you something you needed, how receptive would you be to them?
(g) Does this way of walking remind you of any particular scene (on television, at the theatre or in a certain area of life)?

Clean your palette by literally shaking your body as if shaking off water.

Exercise B

Now, again without altering the position of your head, walk around with the feeling that the roof of your mouth is closer to the ceiling than to the ground, for three minutes. Go down the same list of questions and observe the differences in your response.

The general response to Exercise A is shallow breathing, tunnel vision, a feeling of heaviness and depression, lack of awareness of others and the environment, lack of spontaneity and a slower pace. People often report the similarity of this disposition to that of a prison.

The response to Exercise B is quite different. There are reports of deeper breathing, broader perspective, a feeling of lightness and joy, interest in others and the environment, more spontaneous expression, and a faster pace. The reason for the divergent responses is quite simple. Our thinking and our bodies are intimately linked.

In both cases, nothing in your life was different. You still had the same responsibilities, the same problems, the same bills to pay, the same things you enjoy doing. Your attitude – your relationship with yourself – is the only thing that changed. With a little willpower and concentration we can turn this into a way of life. When we can stay in touch with the impact of our attitudes we wake up to our potential. Our awareness becomes expanded. We become conscious. After all, there *is* no time like the present.

Beauty: When the Other Dancer is the Self

Alice Walker

It is a bright summer day in 1947. My father, a fat, funny man with beautiful eyes and a subversive wit, is trying to decide which of his eight children he will take with him to the county fair. My mother, of course, will not go. She is knocked out from getting most of us ready: I hold my neck stiff against the pressure of her knuckles as she hastily completes the braiding and then beribboning of my hair.

My father is the driver for the rich old white lady up the road. Her name is Miss Mey. She owns all the land for miles around, as well as the house in which we live. All I remember about her is that she once offered to pay my mother 35 cents for cleaning her house, raking up piles of her magnolia leaves, and washing her family's clothes, and that my mother – she of no money, eight children, and a chronic earache – refused it. But I do not think of this in 1947. I am two and a half years old. I want to go everywhere my daddy goes. I am excited at the prospect of riding in a car. Someone has told me fairs are fun. That there is room in the car for only three of us doesn't faze me at all. Whirling happily in my starchy frock, showing off my biscuit-polished patent-leather shoes and lavender socks, tossing my head in a way that makes my ribbons bounce, I stand, hands on hips, before my father. 'Take me, Daddy,' I say with assurance; 'I'm the prettiest!'

Later, it does not surprise me to find myself in Miss Mey's shiny black car, sharing the back seat with the other lucky ones. Does not surprise me that I thoroughly enjoy the fair. At home that night I tell the unlucky ones all I can remember about the merry-go-round, the man who eats live chickens, and the teddy bears, until they say: that's enough, baby Alice. Shut up now, and go to sleep.

It is Easter Sunday, 1950. I am dressed in a green, flocked, scalloped-hem dress (handmade by my adoring sister, Ruth) that has its own smooth satin petticoat and tiny hot-pink roses tucked into each scallop. My shoes, new T-strap patent leather, again highly biscuit-polished. I am six years old and have learned one of the longest Easter speeches to be heard that day, totally unlike the speech I said when I was two: 'Easter lilies/ pure and white/ blossom in/ the morning light.' When I rise to give my speech I do so on a great wave of love and pride and expectation. People in church stop rustling their new crinolines. They seem to hold their breath. I can tell they admire my dress, but it is my spirit, bordering on sassiness (womanishness), they secretly applaud.

'That girl's a little *mess*,' they whisper to each other, pleased.

Naturally I say my speech without stammer or pause, unlike those who stutter, stammer or worst of all, forget. This is before the word 'beautiful' exists in people's vocabulary, but 'Oh, isn't she the *cutest* thing!' frequently floats my way. 'And got so much sense!' they gratefully add . . . for which thoughtful addition I thank them to this day.

It was great fun being cute. But then one day, it ended.

I am eight years old and a tomboy. I have a cowboy hat, cowboy boots, checkered shirt and pants, all red. My playmates are my brothers, two and four years older than I.

Their colours are black and green, the only difference in the way we are dressed. On Saturday nights we all go to the picture show, even my mother; Westerns are her favourite kind of movie. Back home, 'on the ranch', we pretend we are Tom Mix, Hopalong Cassidy, Lash LaRue (we've even named one of our four dogs Lash LaRue); we chase each other for hours rustling cattle, being outlaws, delivering damsels from distress. Then my parents decide to buy my brothers guns. These are not 'real' guns. They shoot 'BBs', copper pellets my brothers say will kill birds. Because I am a girl, I do not get a gun. Instantly I am relegated to the position of Indian. Now there appears a great distance between us. They shoot and shoot at everything with their new guns. I try to keep up with my bow and arrows.

One day while I am standing on top of our makeshift 'garage' – pieces of tin nailed across some poles – holding my bow and arrow and looking out toward the fields, I feel an incredible blow in my right eye. I look down just in time to see my brother lower his gun.

Both brothers rush to my side. My eye stings, and I cover it with my hand. 'If you tell,' they say, 'we will get a whipping. You don't want that to happen, do you?' I do not. 'Here is a piece of wire,' says the older brother, picking it up from the roof; 'say you stepped on one end of it and the other flew up and hit you.' The pain is beginning to start. 'Yes,' I say. 'Yes, I will say that is what happened.' If I do not say this is what happened, I know my brothers will find ways to make me wish I had. But now I will say anything that gets me to my mother.

Confronted by our parents we stick to the lie agreed upon. They place me on a bench on the porch and I close my left eye while they examine the right. There is a tree growing from underneath the porch that climbs past the railing to the roof. It is the last thing my right eye sees. I watch as its trunk, its branches, and then its leaves are blotted out by the rising blood.

241

I am in shock. First there is intense fever, which my father tries to break using lily leaves bound around my head. Then there are chills: my mother tries to get me to eat soup. Eventually, I do not know how, my parents learn what has happened. A week after the 'accident' they take me to see a doctor. 'Why did you wait so long to come?' he asks, looking into my eye and shaking his head. 'Eyes are sympathetic,' he says. 'If one is blind, the other will likely become blind too.'

This comment of the doctor's terrifies me. But it is really how I look that bothers me most. Where the BB pellet struck there is a glob of whitish scar tissue, a hideous cataract, on my eye. Now when I stare at people – a favourite pastime, up to now – they will stare back. Not at the 'cute' little girl, but at her scar. For six years I do not stare at anyone, because I do not raise my head.

Years later, in the throes of a mid-life crisis, I ask my mother and sister whether I changed after the 'accident'. 'No,' they say, puzzled. 'What do you mean?'

What do I mean?

I am eight, and, for the first time, doing poorly in school, where I have been something of a whiz since I was four. We have just moved to the place where the 'accident' occurred. We do not know any of the people around us because this is a different country. The only time I see the friends I knew is when we go back to our old church. The new school is the former state penitentiary. It is a large stone building, cold and draughty, crammed to overflowing with boisterous, ill-disciplined children. On the third floor there is a huge circular imprint of some partition that has been torn out.

'What used to be here?' I ask a sullen girl next to me on our way past it to lunch.

'The electric chair,' says she.

At night I have nightmares about the electric chair, and about all the people reputedly 'fried' in it. I am afraid of the school, where all the students seem to be budding criminals.

'What's the matter with your eye?' they ask, critically.

When I don't answer (I cannot decide whether it was an 'accident' or not), they shove me, insist on a fight.

My brother, the one who created the story about the wire, comes to my rescue. But then brags so much about 'protecting' me, I become sick.

After months of torture at the school, my parents decide to send me back to our old community, to my old school. I live with my grandparents and the teacher they board. But there is no room for Phoebe, my cat. By the time my grandparents decide there *is* room and I ask for my cat, she cannot be found. Miss Yarborough, the boarding teacher, takes me under her wing, and begins to teach me to play the piano. But soon she marries an African – a 'prince,' she says – and is whisked away to his continent.

At my old school there is at least one teacher who loves me. She is the teacher who 'knew me before I was born' and bought my first baby clothes. It is she who makes life bearable. It is her presence that finally helps me turn on the one child at the school who continually calls me 'one-eyed bitch'. One day I simply grab him by his coat and beat him until I am satisfied. It is my teacher who tells me my mother is ill.

My mother is lying in bed in the middle of the day, something I have never seen. She is in too much pain to speak. She has an abscess in her ear. I stand looking down on her, knowing that if she dies, I cannot live. She is being treated with warm oils and hot bricks held against her cheek. Finally a doctor comes. But I must go back to my grandparents' house. The weeks pass but I am hardly aware of it. All I know is that my mother might die, my father is not so jolly, my brothers still have their guns, and I am the one sent away from home.

'You did not change,' they say.

Did I imagine the anguish of never looking up?

I am twelve. When relatives come to visit I hide in my room. My cousin Brenda, just my age, whose father works in the post office and whose mother is a nurse, comes to find me. 'Hello,' she says. And then she asks, looking at my recent school picture, which I did not want taken, and on which the 'glob', as I think of it, is clearly visible, 'You still can't see out of that eye?'

'No,' I say, and flop back on the bed over my book.

That night, as I do almost every night, I abuse my eye. I rant and rave at it, in front of the mirror. I plead with it to clear up before morning. I tell it I hate and despise it. I do not pray for sight. I pray for beauty.

'You did not change,' they say.

I am fourteen and baby-sitting for my brother Bill, who lives in Boston. He is my favourite brother and there is a strong bond between us. Understanding my feelings of shame and ugliness he and his wife take me to a local hospital, where the 'glob' is removed by a doctor named O. Henry. There is still a small bluish crater where the scar tissue was, but the ugly white stuff is gone. Almost immediately I become a different person from the girl who does not raise her head. Or so I think. Now that I've raised my head I win the boyfriend of my dreams. Now that I've raised my head I have plenty of friends. Now that I've raised my head classwork comes from my lips as faultlessly as Easter speeches did, and I leave high school as valedictorian, most popular student, and *queen*, hardly believing my luck. Ironically, the girl who was voted most beautiful in our class (and was) was later shot twice through the chest by a male companion, using a 'real' gun, while she was pregnant. But that's another story in itself. Or is it?

'You did not change,' they say.

244

It is now thirty years since the 'accident'. A beautiful journalist comes to visit and to interview me. She is going to write a cover story for her magazine that focuses on my latest book. 'Decide how you want to look on the cover,' she says. 'Glamorous, or whatever.'

Never mind 'glamorous', it is the 'whatever' that I hear. Suddenly all I can think of is whether I will get enough sleep the night before the photography session: if I don't, my eye will be tired and wander as blind eyes will.

At night in bed with my lover I think up reasons why I should not appear on the cover of a magazine. 'My meanest critics will say I've sold out,' I say. 'My family will now realise I write scandalous books.'

'But what's the real reason you don't want to do this?' he asks.

'Because in all probability,' I say in a rush, 'my eye won't be straight.'

'It will be straight enough,' he says. Then, 'Besides, I thought you'd made your peace with that.'

And I suddenly remember that I have.

I remember:

I am talking to my brother Jimmy, asking if he remembers anything unusual about the day I was shot. He does not know I consider that day the last time my father, with his sweet home remedy of cool lily leaves, chose me, and that I suffered and raged inside because of this. 'Well,' he says, 'all I remember is standing by the side of the highway with Daddy, trying to flag down a car. A white man stopped, but when Daddy said he needed somebody to take his little girl to the doctor, he drove off.'

I remember:

I am in the desert for the first time. I fall totally in love with it. I am so overwhelmed by its beauty, I confront for the first time, consciously, the meaning of the doctor's words years ago. 'Eyes are sympathetic. If one is blind, the other will likely become blind too.' I realise I have dashed about the world madly, looking at this, looking at that, storing up images against the fading of the light. *But I might have missed seeing the desert!* The shock of that possibility – and gratitude for over twenty-five years of sight – sends me literally to my knees. Poem after poem comes – which is perhaps how poets pray.

> *On Sight*
> I am so thankful I have seen
> The Desert
> And the creatures in the desert
> And the desert itself.
>
> The desert has its own moon
> Which I have seen
> With my own eye.
> There is no flag on it.
>
> Trees of the desert have arms
> All of which are always up
> That is because the moon is up
> The sun is up
> Also the sky
> The stars
> Clouds
> None with flags.
>
> If there *were* flags, I doubt
> the trees would point.
> Would you?

But mostly, I remember this:

I am twenty-seven, and my baby daughter is almost three. Since her birth I have worried about her discovery that her mother's eyes are different from other people's. Will she be embarrassed? I think. What will she say? Every day she watches a television programme called *Big Blue Marble*. It begins with a picture of the earth as it appears from the moon. It is bluish, a little battered-looking, but full of light, with whitish clouds swirling around it. Every time I see it I weep with love, as if it is a picture of Grandma's house. One day when I am putting Rebecca down for her nap, she suddenly focuses on my eye. Something inside me cringes, gets ready to try to protect myself. All children are cruel about physical differences, I know from experience, and that they don't always mean to be is another matter. I assume Rebecca will be the same.

But no-o-o. She studies my face intently as we stand, her inside and me outside her crib. She even holds my face maternally between her dimpled little hands. Then, looking every bit as serious and lawyerlike as her father, she says, as if it may just possibly have slipped my attention: 'Mommy, there's a *world* in your eye.' (As in, 'Don't be alarmed, or do anything crazy.') And then, gently, but with great interest: 'Mommy, where did you *get* that world in your eye?'

For the most part, the pain left then. (So what, if my brothers grew up to buy even more powerful pellet guns for their sons and to carry real guns themselves. So what, if a young 'Morehouse man' once nearly fell off the steps of Trevor Arnett Library because he thought my eyes were blue.) Crying and laughing I ran to the bathroom, while Rebecca mumbled and sang herself off to sleep. Yes indeed, I realised, looking into the mirror. There *was* a world in my eye. And I saw that it was possible to love it: that in fact, for all it had taught me of shame and anger and inner vision, I *did* love it. Even to see it drifting out of orbit in boredom, or rolling up out of fatigue, not to mention floating back at attention in excitement (bearing witness, a friend has called it), deeply suitable to my personality and even characteristic of me.

That night I dream I am dancing to Stevie Wonder's song 'Always' (the name of the song is really 'As', but I hear it as 'Always'). As I dance, whirling and joyous, happier than I've ever been in my life, another bright-faced dancer joins me. We dance and kiss each other and hold each other through the night. The other dancer has obviously come through all right, as I have done. She is beautiful, whole and free. And she is also me.

Black Old Age . . .
The Diaspora of the Senses?

Beryl Gilroy

I am thinking about my being black and growing old in Britain. Will my old age, I wonder, be a calamitous plunge deeper into the underclass, or simply part of the general heritage of the struggling old, regardless of race or class?

Some white old people face old age with resentment. They are, however, part of the dominant tribe, and when push turns to shove they will assuredly be taken care of against all comers.

Everything is valid in the fight with the ravages of old age. Implants, cosmetic surgery, hair transplants, dyes and other concoctions are part of the confrontation between body and time. Most of this is beyond the reach of the poor and aged black, so old age has its way with us.

For most of us, death can be both sudden and close, and so reaching the allotted lifespan of three score years and ten is a time of rejoicing and pleasure. However, in this society only youth is given validity. It does not matter how efficient or committed a woman has been in her working life. On her sixtieth birthday and retirement she is assumed to have undergone some comprehensive deterioration. Experience becomes irrelevant to future generations who need to learn. Knowledge built up over a lifetime is thrown away, and senility and mental sterility are thought to have been acquired in quantity.

Western societies have developed various ways of casting aside the lives of the old. Let us therefore look, and only very briefly, at our African heritage prior to the cult of the gun, famine, drought and economic destabilisation. We must not forget the machinations of the multinationals or the part played by the trading nations in the destruction of African cultural values, with more vigour since so many gained independence. The culture contained an ideology of old age which was taken to the West Indies by the slaves, who restructured it. There were no bona fide family members for committed care. No age-grouped members of the gender rituals like circumcision. Therefore kitchen communism, community care, societies and begotten or adopted children ensured care for the aged. The explicit tenets of responsibility for the old, made indigent by neglect, overwork and cruelty, were thus maintained.

African old age brought ancestral spirits through custom, behaviour and ritual into the lives of both young and old. Life allowed rebirth of the dead time after time to bring back the wisdom of the sages.

Old age marked the passing of time and it was time alone that allowed the harvesting of wisdom which permitted the advising of others. Living life co-ordinated moments of time and space.

True, today technologies have ensured that all old people have time on their hands, but there is not always the will or the resources to bring zest to endeavour. We are patronised by word and gesture and given minimal thought in the distribution of resources.

Black old people – men mostly – appear only briefly on TV. The grandfather in *EastEnders* tries desperately to give reality to the pointless part he plays. And the old man in the *Why Pay More?* ad is as stereotypic as ever as he shouts his unconcern with helping his wife to the viewing world.

Like the true black stereotype he has found a warm place to sit down and be busy. The woman is a shrieking voice – ignored by her man and addressed as 'woman'.

In old age we no longer run for cover from the racists of society, but we remain vulnerable. Some seek us out at election time. We are visible only then, for they are seeking power through politics. Promises! Promises! Promises! Forget them. During the long day we shop a little, walk to the park, feed the ducks, and look at the photographs with all their memories. There is no need to hurry back home. You are alone. The children have grown up and flown the nest. They visit when they can, and when they can, provide extra necessities. Your partner too has been lost to time.

> As sweet youth fades
> And age weaves its cobwebs
> Into limbs and hair and lively life,
> We wonder what rare metaphor will come
> After the dancing years, the loving time,
> The labouring time
> The body-for-others time,
> And we look back and rake the past
> And ramble over thorns and roses
> Seeking those who were with us then.

So I thought while I was waiting for my bus. It did not come but the piles of chewing-gum so liberally strewn upon the pavement stuck to my shoes and made me wonder at its cause. My bus still had not come several minutes later, but a 'sister' I had not seen before approached me. She was over the middle-age mark and neatly dressed in mourning. She spoke to me softly, at first, and then suddenly she released the tensions in her throat in a strangled scream.

'Me affe tell you,' she said. 'Me husban, he dead. He

electrocute last week. The good Lord take 'im. I miss 'im. I miss 'im so much me head going mad.'

As she spoke even the pores on her face dripped tears. Her body had become a graveyard of sadness and disconsolation. Her movements too, showed anger and grief running through them like a thick cord, lassoing me to her need. I could find nothing appropriate to say to this stranger, bound to me only by colour, but she took me by the hand and led me to her flat around the corner.

By now my bus had come and gone, so I sat and listened as she poured out her torment, her loneliness and her pain. She talked of the empty hours she could not now fill, the changes she knew she must make. I listened as I had never done before, and as the hours passed I wished that I could stay with her, for what she needed most was another of her kind.

From whichever island of the Caribbean she had come, she would have been surrounded by her friends and relatives at home. As a woman sick with grief she would be tended and cared for. Words from the Good Book would be offered for comfort and spiritual presence, and in a final effort to give up feelings of loss and accept that the spirit of the person had passed on, the women would gather on the ninth day after the burial, and by rhythmic clapping and singing woo her into dancing away her grief in the Ritual Nine Night Wake.

This was usual in the village in which I grew up. Ritual was important. At funerals women carried well-worked wreaths of twigs and dried flowers to celebrate the passing of the old, and children carried green branches when the young passed away.

Now there was this old black woman all alone. A solitary widow. 'Few black people live round here,' she said. 'So near the depot. So near the trains. We had no choice.' Like mine her widowhood was sudden and owned only by herself. 'God never gave me children.'

They could not all gather around to channel away her pain. For her, only the church existed. Her grief underlined the seeking, the searching for a better life that is immigration, and which sometimes leads to isolation and despair. She was content to sit and quietly clutch her memories, and show me her photographs of a life I could not imagine, with a man I could never now know. But she had her quota of laughter and 'Laugh stories' and the myths, proverbs and dreams that kept our forebears sane in slavery and which now comforted her. 'Tank God I can remember,' she said. 'We must all open our eyes to memory. He did good mostly. Nothing tempted him too far.'

How right she had been about memory. It is able to double-take, leave out, accentuate and change. It brings together mind, body and brain. We can wear it like an extra jumper in the winter or like a sunshade in the summer. We can do what we like with the chameleon of memory.

Memory begins before words appear. As babies we recognise those we love through touch and smell. Memory helps us know what goes on inside us before we are able to speak. Edmund Gosse, an English writer, tells an incredible story in his autobiography. It shows the power of memory. He was all alone in his high chair while he waited for the family to arrive for lunch. Their pet, a large and greedy dog, dashed in from the garden and carried off the leg of lamb which was to be served. He could not tell what had happened to the meat because he had not yet learned how to talk. Many years later when the incident once more surfaced he was able to explain the fate of the meat by recalling the buried memory.

Memory can provide the oil that is poured upon troubled waters, or stoke smoking fires to flame. Memory is a child of the guts and the emotion, of the brain and the heart and the lips. It is the dresser of time – in silks or satins or bruising flax which our forefathers wore during the diaspora. Memory makes us laugh and cry in turn. We cannot escape it.

Black communities on the whole take responsibility for their old and their elderly parents but this can be changed by the pressure of distance, unemployment and illness. These are different times. Boys no longer feel it their duty to look after their mothers, and in order for the women to do so, they must themselves work and leave the children to grandparents, already worn out by lived life. We must find the skill, patience and endurance to cope with the young and so allow ourselves to be trapped in the historical role. We are living longer, and as a consequence are discovering lots of exciting things to do. We are asking questions about the roles we play and what we need out of this life which is hardly a rehearsal for a better one here on earth. My friend, recently retired, has rejected traditional roles of baby-sitting and child-watching and opened a health shop for the elderly. She is enjoying many wonderful moments.

Yet it is not an all-or-nothing relationship between us and our grandchildren. Most grandchildren eulogise their grandparents and understand when they do not want to be the main care-giver. Many of us keep enlightened contact with our grandchildren by refusing to buy into their affections, and by never supporting the consumer-monster activities at which so many young people excel. Like them we enjoy life, or strive to, but we think of death and they do not.

Death is the truth that divides the old from the young who think that they are indestructible and say so. And since only the old readily and easily die, there is guarded affiliation between youth and old age. When my grand-daughter said, referring to us, her grandmothers, her mother and herself, 'There are two old ladies. One young mother and one little girl,' I felt troubled. I had never been described as that before.

Segregation by age is something I have yet to get used to. Life and its times were for everyone in my village. Everyone had fun. The silly fun and the sensible fun.

I can remember when I encountered the word 'baby-sitter', wondering what it was. The closest was 'nurse', and children with nurses had no mothers, we believed. There was never any parcelling out of people into sections and groups. Old age meant respect, regard and consideration. Today the culture is global and led by America with all its light and shade, its preference for whiteness and the associations it gives to it. Americans are generous people, giving what is needed and what is not to the poor. What is of no use in the developed countries, or is merely self-indulgence, is freely offered as aid to the underdeveloped peoples of the world. The other day a 71-year-old grand-mother who had just returned from one of the 'aided countries' told me how a Teddy bear of enormous size nearly gave her relation a heart attack. 'Nobody knew what to do with it. An ugly ting like dat. The man push it to the child and kept on saying "Teddy bear, Teddy bear" and kissing it. But we never trust it because it could turn magic when the white man went home.' Affluence can be the father of ignorance.

This is a strange society; stranger still is the rest of the world. It made us – the patient, providing mother – dispensable. The children are a gift to life as old age would make us a gift to death. Yet life has validated us as mother, wife and friend. Thoughts of the past occupy our minds but the past has gone. Whatever its colour, we cannot retrieve its texture or its momentum. We have gained and lost.

Practically, we have gained personal freedom, peace of mind and the right to an individual identity. We are our-selves without encroachment from family or community. We are given an extra £10 at Christmas and receive it with as much unconcern as your forebears received their extra rations of flour, corn and salted beef in the bad old days, also at Christmas. We agree that £10 is the bounty of a caring government or a loving social worker. There are other concessions too – like the annual gift of a pound of butter from the EC. But we must know the venue and wear spurs on our elbows. Old age is and can design impoverishment as well as self-sufficiency. An inadequate pension, for example, can generate its own kind of poverty trap.

My most prized concession is my bus pass – a cold dark green this year. A proportion of my poll tax has been recycled to pay for it. It is not really free! Nor is the eye test which so many of us need. According to the minister it should cost £10, but the optician's secretary assures me that the minister meant from £10, and demands another four. But no matter. I have my bus pass which I highly prize. It *is* a cold dark green this year and my poll tax *has* helped to pay for it, so true to old age I repeat myself.

I catch the 10a.m. bus – the 'Geriatrics Express', as it is called – and find nubile women and burly males (school students I presume) looped around the seats set aside for the elderly or the handicapped. Black or white, they watch the 'Shrinklies', as we are described, lurch about as we stand, grasping for support in the speeding bus, and gasping with the effort. When the lurching stops and someone can recover enough to ask one of those compassionate youngsters, 'Are you old or handicapped?', their guilty smiles even turn to laughter.

Life has taught them to sit and watch. We also watch. What do we see? We see that some of our young black people have lost cultural respect for old age and the ability to recognise the needs of the aged. The past means nothing to them. All responses are generated by their present. Some of these young people have learned neither faith, nor hope, nor charity in our affluent society. Love and loving are sexual mores to them, as their rap, so-ca and other musics decree.

For us, to work was to love. Work wove the threads of effort into experience – a tangible thing, which once saved us as a race from extermination. As women, experience helped us towards resistance to people who attacked those wisdoms we once knew – wisdoms of people who overcame all efforts to destroy us as wives, mothers and workers. We were able to love then, and continue to do so now. We have shown this quality in all that we have been asked to do. Today even work has died on us.

Old age celebrates our ability to survive, and eventually comes to a place where we can be grandmothers with gentleness and certainty. For black women, life with all its spikes and its countless thorns has always been lived. Will our old age be yet another diaspora? The diaspora of the senses?

Have no fear. We won't let that happen. We would not let ourselves be discarded, abandoned or left to fall into the pits of life like sediment.

We resolve

to keep as active as we can;
to treat each day of life after three-score and ten as a gift;
to share, to love, to affirm;
to create in ourselves all that is joyous;
to know and enjoy the intangibles of creation – such as valour and sacrifice.

We are a whole people. We have survived. And when the years pass and everyone else has succumbed to mindless change, we shall be the same. Black.

Contributors

....

Patricia Joy Agana is a mother of four children and a grandmother. She was born in Hackney in 1954, of a Jamaican mother and Nigerian father and is the eldest of six children. She has worked in the voluntary sector for twenty-four years seventeen of which have been spent working with children. The past seven years she has spent developing a free counselling service for who adult women have suffered childhood sexual assault and a support service for professionals working in the field, this includes advice and supervision. During the last five years through her own consultancy, Training for Life, Patricia has been contracted in to help devise, advise and train on Brent and Lambeth Social Services child protection courses. Also, she has provided consultancy to residential childcare institutions. Patricia Agana conceived of and cordinated the conference in 1991, Black Women Living and Working with Child Sexual Assault.

Elizabeth N. Anionwu worked as a health visitor and community nurse tutor in Brent between 1971 and 1977. In 1979 she helped to set up the first sickle cell counselling centre in Britain based in Brent. She was head of the centre until 1990, when she left to become a lecturer in community genetic counselling at the Institute of Child Health, University of London.

Nozipho P. January-Bardill has had a background in Education and has taught in Southern Africa and England at Secondary, Further Education and Tertiary Levels. She has worked as an independent Management and Training consultant for local, national and international organisations in the public and voluntary sectors, in the fields of Equal Opportunities

259

policies and practices; race and gender equality in the workplace; organisational analysis; management practice and HIV/AIDS. Her work in HIV/AIDS focused on the needs of black communities in Britain. She is a founder member of the Black HIV and AIDS Network. Nozipho has recently returned to live and work in South Africa.

Sheridan Burton is a senior home care organiser for a London borough. She is also a mother, qualified nurse and adult foster carer and, like most women, a home manager. She has worked to improve the quality of home care for black clients. She is at heart, an 'artist in waiting'. She was a founder member of Camden and Islington Black Sisters.

Antoinette Clark was a research and policy development officer for Rights of Women, a feminist legal project which provides advice and support. She is also committed to researching and writing on issues which affect the lives of women and children, particularly black women. This article is for her daughter Kalli Clark-Sternberg.

Angela Davis is a teacher, author, lecturer and internationally recognised social activist. She teaches philosophy, aesthetics and women's studies at San Francisco State University and the San Francisco Art Institute. She is author of several books.

Shamis Dirir is a Somali and came to Britain in 1967. She has always been interested in health education, particalarly women's health. In 1979 she set up the Somali Women's Association and in early 1980 she founded the Somali Community and Cultural Association, in 1982 she organised the London Black Women's Health Action Project to campaign against Female Genital Mutilation.

Jenny Douglas is director of health promotion for Sandwell Health Authority. She is African-Caribbean and has worked in the field of health promotion for a number of years. She has also been involved in a number of community health initiatives, both locally and nationally, and is at present involved with a number of research projects on the health needs and experiences of black and minority ethnic communities in Sandwell.

Paula Thomas Fenton suffers from lupus. She has campaigned to increase awareness of lupus as a disease which can affect African-Caribbean and Asian women. She is founder of Luton and District Lupus Group.

Sula Thomas Forero is originally from West Africa – part Sierra-Leonean, part Yoruba. Born in London and raised in Kent, she moved to London in the mid-1970s, where she began a seven year varied work experience in London and Europe. This included four years in the performing arts. In the mid-1980s Sula began health related studies. She holds a national diploma in physical therapies and qualifications in bodywork. She is a practising and developing bodywork practitioner with a strong interest in traditional medicine and healing. Fot the past five years she has worked as a freelance bodywork practitioner – practising and teaching in the health service and in private practice in Clapham, South London.

Beryl Gilroy was a student in England in the early 1950s. She was the first black woman appointed as a teacher in London; and the first to write culture-based school texts about Caribbean life. She became the only black principal of Beckford School in Camden. She has written a number of children's books, her autobiography, *Black Teacher*; two novellas, *Frangipani House* and *Boy-Sandwich*; and a collection of poetry, *Echoes and Voices*. Her most recent book, *Stedman and Joanna – A Love in Bondage: Dedicated Love in the Eighteenth Century*, is historical fiction set in England, Surinam and the Netherlands.

Jewelle L. Gomez has written for numerous publications including the *New York Times*, the *Village Voice*, *Essence* and *Belles Lettres*. She is the author of two collections of poetry. Her novel, *The Gilda Stories*, was published by Sheba Feminist Publishers in 1991.

Zora Neale Hurston has written several books including *Dust Tracks on the Road, Jonah's Gourd Vine* and *Their Eyes Were Watching God* (all published by Virago). She died in 1960.

Leonora Kane is a social worker. She currently works as a lecturer in further education with social care students and managers. She has raised two children who have flowered into sophisticated political thinkers. She is a founder member of Camden and Islington Black Sisters, and has been involved in many local, national and international political campaigns.

Audre Lorde was a black lesbian, poet, mother, warrior woman, feminist, essayist, novelist and educator and political campaigner. She died in St Croix Virgin Islands in November, 1992, at the age of 58.

Ann Phoenix teaches psychology in the Department of Human Sciences, Brunel University. The research on which this paper is based was done at the Thomas Coram Research Unit, Institute of Education, University of London.

Dr. Khaleghl Quinn is author of three definitive books on self-preservation – *Stand Your Ground, Reclaim Your Power,* and *Art of Self-Defence* – and presented a long-running television series on the subject. Her pioneering work has taken self-defence away from its traditional perception and into a balanced blend of effective physical techniques and confident self assurance.

A world-acknowledged martial arts expert and Chi Kung master, Khaleghl teaches at her Quindo Centre in North London.

Barbara Smith is one of the leading activists in the feminist movement and editor/author of numerous works. Her literary criticism, reviews and essays have appeared in scores of publications including the *New York Times*. She edited *Home Girls: A Black Feminist Anthology* and is a co-founder and publisher of Kitchen Table: Women of Color Press.

Protasia Torkington was born in South Africa in 1940.
She trained as a state registered nurse, and as a midwife.
After coming to England in 1968, she specialised in paediatrics.
Subsequently she took A levels and obtained a degree in
sociology. She is a Fellow of Liverpool University and is a
senior lecturer in sociology at Liverpool Institute of Higher
Education. She has been particularly involved in and concerned
with health and race issues.

Alice Walker is a distinguished American writer, author of
numerous volumes of fiction, poetry, essays and short stories.
In 1983 she won both the Pulitzer Prize and the American
Book Award for her novel *The Color Purple* (Harcourt
Brace Jovanovich and The Women's Press, 1982). The book
was subsequently made into an Oscar-nominated feature
film.

Melba Wilson is a freelance journalist who writes on health
and social affairs. Her book, *Crossing the Boundary – Black
Women Survive Incest* was published by Virago Press in 1993.

List of organisations

....

Women and Sickle Cell Disorders,
Elizabeth N. Anionwu
Sickle Cell Society
54 Station Road
Harlesden
London NW10 4UB
Tel: (081) 961 7795/8346

Organisation for Sickle Cell Anaemia Research (OSCAR)
Sickle Cell Community Centre
Tiverton Road
Tottenham
London N15 6RT
Tel: (081) 802 3055/0944

Addresses and telephone numbers of National Health Service
sickle cell counselling centres can be obtained by sending a
stamped addressed envelope to:

   Dr Elizabeth N. Anionwu
   Department of Clinical Genetics
   Institute of Child Health
   30 Guildford Street
   London WC1N 1EH

One Woman's Experience of Lupus
Paula Thomas Fenton

Resources: Britain
Luton & District Lupus Group
c/o Paula Thomas
19 High Mead
Luton, Beds
LU3 1RY
Tel: (0582) 504785

Dr Evonne von Heussen-Contryman
Specialist Genetic Diseases
31 Radford Road
Royal Leamington Spa
Warwicks CV31 1NF
Tel: (0926) 338622

Claudia Jones Organisation
103 Stoke Newington Road
London N16 8BX
Tel: (071) 241 1646

New group for sufferers being set up by:
Brenda and Angela Jackson
49 Leighton Road
Enfield
Tel: (081) 366 9746

Note: None of these self-help groups is able to help anxious sufferers. There is a definite need for training.

The Arthritis & Rheumatism Council
Copeman House
St Mary's Court
St Mary's Gate
Chesterfield,
Derbyshire S41 7TD
Tel: (0246) 558033

Resources: United States
Lupus Foundation of America, Inc.
1717 Massachusetts Avenue NW
Washington, DC 20036
Tel: (202) 328 4550
or (800) 558 0121

References and further reading
The Black Women's Health Book – Speaking for Ourselves, ed.
Evelyn C. White, Seal Press, 1990.
    3131 Western Avenue
    Suite 410
    Seattle, Washington 98121

The Lambeth Women and Children's Health Project: Working with Child Sexual Assault
Patricia Joy Agana

On 14 February 1990 Lambeth Women and Children's Health
Project held a conference entitled 'Black Women Living and
Working with the Effects of Child Sexual Assault'. Drawing
from the historical experience of the work done by women
survivors of childhood sexual assault, the conference was the
first of its kind in the country in that it provided a forum for
professionals and survivors, the statutory and voluntary sectors,
as well as facilitating debate between women of African, Asian,
Caribbean and Chinese descent. The aim was to create a
forum where the issues relating to our communities were at
least being discussed by us first, so that we could make

informed decisions about matters that had hitherto been decided on our behalf.

Lambeth Women and Children's Health Project provides counselling information and support to all women, having due respect for race, culture, age, sexuality and ability. We are particularly interested in developing resources for people of African Caribbean and Asian descent and in creating self-reliance amongst those who are culturally, socially and politically disadvantaged.

Lambeth Women and Children's Health Project may be contacted at:

> Angel Town Estate
> Hollis House
> Unit 8
> London SW9
> *Tel*: (071) 737 7151

A Needle in a Haystack: Finding Support as a Survivor of Domestic Violence
Antoinette Clark

Citizens' Advice Bureau   Look under Citizens' Advice Bureau in the phone book or ring the London headquarters on (071) 251 2000. For the rest of the country ring (071) 833 2181.

Department of Social Security   Look in the phone book under 'Benefits Agency'.

Law Centres Federation   Duchess House 18–19 Warren Street, London W1P 5DB. (071) 387 8570   Will tell you where your nearest law centre is.

Lesbian and Gay Switchboard   24-hour hotline: (071) 837 7324.

London Women's Aid   (071) 251 6537   Emergency number on answerphone. Should also be able to give you contact numbers for Asian women's refuges, Black women's refuges, Latin American Women's Aid.

National Women's Aid   (0272) 428 368. (As for London Women's Aid.)

Rape Crisis   PO Box 69, London WC1X 9NJ   (071) 837 1600.

Rights of Women   Postal and telephone free legal advice service (can recommend feminist solicitors) 52–54 Featherstone Street, London EC1 8RT (071) 251 6577.

Sanctuary Project Provides counselling for women who have been sexually abused. Office number: (071) 371 4666. Counselling line: (071) 371 4333.

Society of Black Lawyers Has a list of Black solicitors and barristers. 444 Brixton Road, London SW9. (071) 737 1060.

Standing Committee on Sexually Abused Children 73 St Charles Square, London W10 6EJ. (081) 969 4808/ (081) 960 6376.

Local advice agencies Ring the town hall. This also applies for addresses and numbers of the local homeless persons units.

Therapeutic Bodywork *Sula Thomas Forero*

The Hoxton Health Group offers a range of bodywork treatments, relaxation classes and other complementary therapies for those over the age of 55 and living in Hackney or City. A registered charity, it charges a £3 per month membership fee which entitles members to the use of all treatments and facilities. There is a waiting list at present. St Leonard's Hospital, Nuttall Street, Hackney, London N1 5LZ *Tel*: (071) 739 2533, Wednesday and Thursday afternoons and Fridays.

The Medical Foundation for the Care of Victims of Torture provides a service for survivors of torture, most of whom are refugees. They offer counselling, psychotherapy and bodywork. There is no charge for the service. 96 Grafton Road, London NW5 3EJ *Tel*: (071) 284 4321.

Sula Thomas Forero can be contacted on (071) 627 5431

Women and Health is run for and by women. It offers quite an extensive range of bodywork treatments, other complementary therapies and health-care facilities for women who live or work in Camden. They operate a sliding scale of fees. 4 Carol Street London NW1 0HU *Tel*: (071) 482 2786.

Women and Medical Practice offers counselling, some bodywork and health advice. They also have a sliding scale of fees. This service is open to all women. 40 Turnpike Lane London N8 0PS *Tel*: (081) 888 2782.

Index

···

CROSSING THE BOUNDARY
Black Women Survive Incest

Melba Wilson

'A valuable work in a myriad of ways . . . Wilson's is a voice full of determination, strength and accessibility' – *The Voice*

This pathbreaking book, written by a survivor, is the culmination of Melba Wilson's long-held desire to write about an experience which has affected her and countless other women and children. Looking at the situation of Black women and incest, she focuses on the costs of that survival and the strengths which sustain it. She writes from the conviction that the taboo against speaking out must be broken, while debunking the myth that incest is the norm in Black communities. Voices of individual women, a discussion of incest in the autobiographical and fictional work of Black writers such as Maya Angelou, Alice Walker and Joan Riley, the role of professionals, and the dynamics of sex and sexual oppression in relation to gender, class and race – all are examined in this brave and important book.

THE HEART OF THE RACE
Black Women's Lives in Britain

Beverley Bryan, Stella Dadzie &
Susanne Scafe

**'A balanced tribute to the undefeated creativity,
resilience and resourcefulness of Black women in
Britain today'** – *Margaret Busby, New Society*

**Winner of the Martin Luther King Memorial Prize
1985**

The Heart of the Race powerfully records what life is like
for Black women in Britain: grandmothers drawn to the
promise of the 'mother country' in the 1950s talk of a
different reality; young girls describe how their
aspirations at school are largely ignored; working women
tell of their commitments to families, jobs, communities.
With clarity and determination, these Afro–Caribbean
women discuss their treatment by the Welfare State, their
housing situations, their health, their self-images – and
their confrontation with the racism they encounter all too
often. Here too is Black women's celebration of their
culture and their struggle to create a new social order in
this country.

HYSTERECTOMY
and the alternatives

Jan Clark

'**A thoroughly researched and practical contribution
to the literature on women's health . . . Any woman
faced with the possibility of a hysterectomy should
read this book in the quietness of her own home, and
encourage her husband or partner to read it too**'
– *Dr Jonathon A. Davis, Consultant Gynaecologist,
Stobhill General Hospital, Glasgow.*

Around 80,000 women undergo a hysterectomy every
year in the UK. But is the operation always necessary?
Many women don't know what is really involved, or that
often there are options other than major surgery. This
book details the entire process from patient complaint to
post–operative recovery. It outlines the many reasons for
the operation, deals sympathetically with the intimate
emotional and physical concerns, offers practical advice
and shares women's profound and courageous
experiences of the trauma. It presents recent
developments within orthodox medicine and explores in
depth whether complementary therapies such as
acupuncture, medical herbalism and homoeopathy offer
viable alternative treatments.

WITH WINGS
An Anthology of Literature by Women with Disabilities

Edited by Marsha Saxton & Florence Howe

'It shouts out our talents, our concerns, with some wonderful pieces of work. In doing so, it claims both a place within the general culture and attempts to change that culture'
– *Jenny Morris, Feminist Review*

With Wings speaks with the many voices of women – young and old, black and white, heterosexual and lesbian, rich and poor – on a common theme. Through personal accounts, fiction and poetry, women describe the experience of physical disability, exploring its effects on their relationships with family, friends and lovers, and reaching out to transcend the barriers of being female and disabled. While dispelling myths and stereotypes, the collection celebrates the strengths and talents of these women and girls, offering a personal look at the fierce rage and pain of physical and social devaluing and the triumph of overcoming them. More than thirty writers, some of them – such as Nancy Mairs, Adrienne Rich, Muriel Rukeyser and Alice Walker – well known, others previously unpublished, capture the striving for dignity, self-expression, love and independence in the day-to-day reality of life for women with disabilities.

MATTERS OF LIFE AND DEATH
Women Speak about AIDS

Edited by Ines Rieder and Patricia Ruppelt

'A sad, wise, kind, brave, necessary book'
– *Angela Carter*

Matters of Life and Death is a remarkable collection of writings by women whose lives have been irrevocably changed by AIDS. We hear the voices of women who have AIDS or who have tested HIV positive; women who have cared for husbands, brothers, lovers, friends and children until their death from AIDS; women who work as prostitutes and as advocates for prostitutes' rights; and women who are AIDS activists in the fields of medicine, education and counselling. They bring home to us the magnitude of the epidemic and the shattering impact AIDS has on people's everyday lives.

This is a book that everyone should read, a book that offers extraordinary insights into our most fundamental preoccupations: love, sexuality, grief and bereavement, society's relation to illness and death.